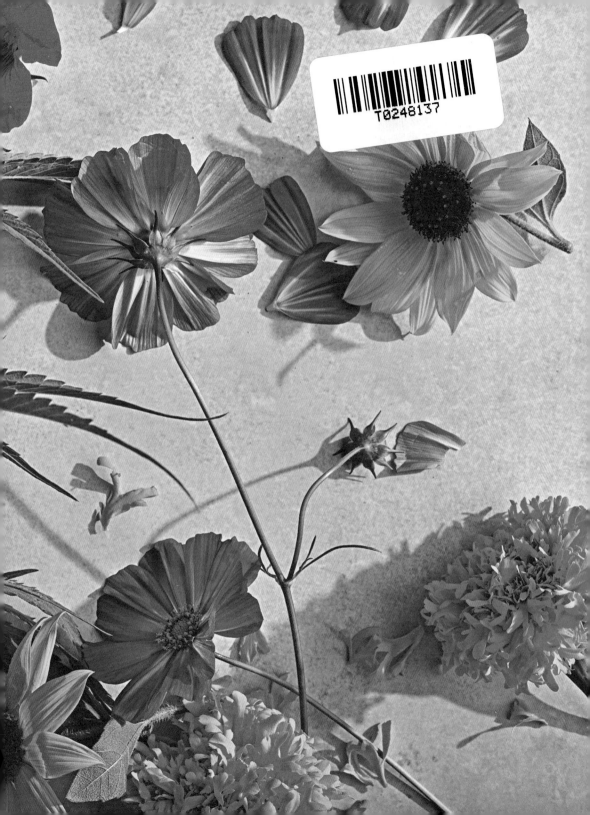

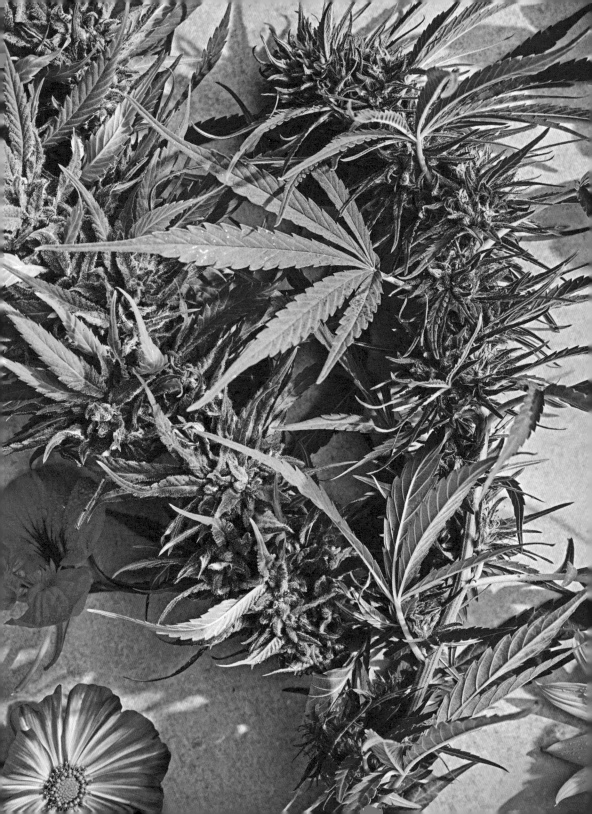

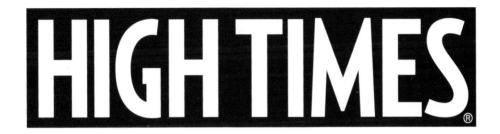

CANNABIS COCKTAILS

SEASONAL SIPS & HIGH TEAS FOR EVERY OCCASION

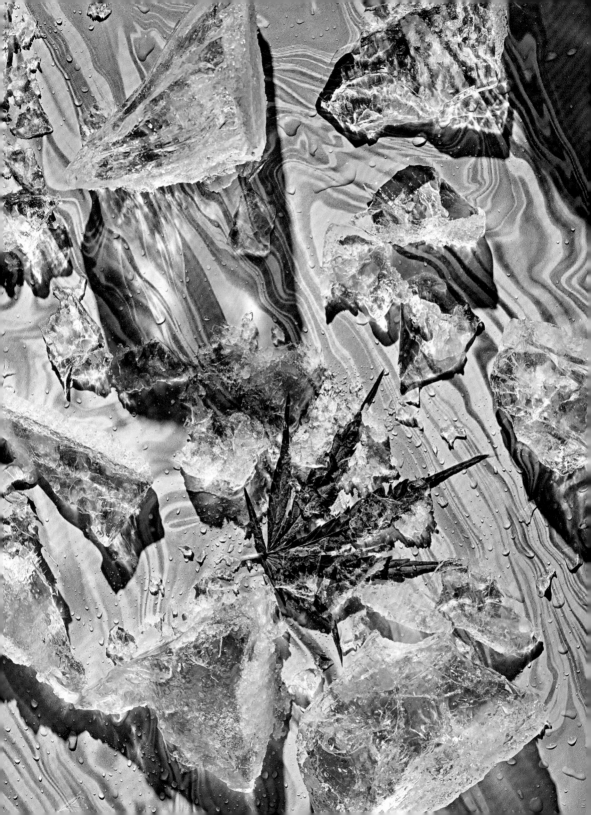

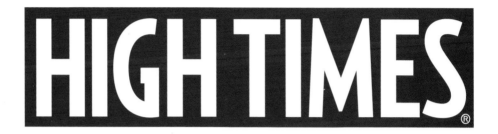

CANNABIS COCKTAILS

SEASONAL SIPS & HIGH TEAS FOR EVERY OCCASION

Jamie Evans

Photography by Eva Kolenko

INSIGHT
EDITIONS

SAN RAFAEL · LOS ANGELES · LONDON

CONTENTS

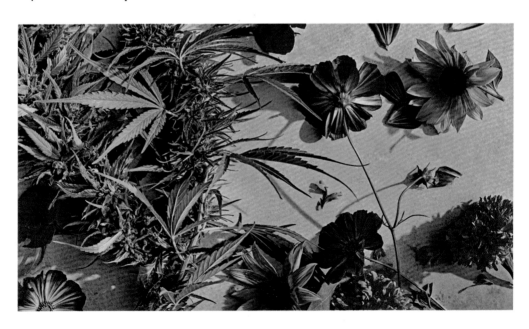

FOREWORD

In the nearly ten years since I wrote the first book on the topic (according to the Library of Congress), named *Cannabis Cocktails, Mocktails & Tonics* (Fair Winds Press, 2016), there haven't been many others writing in this genre. Since then, an entire generation has passed, and there still haven't been many competitors in the cannabis-infused beverage book market that were teaching anything delicious. . . until now.

Most of the books that I've seen are extremely rough takes on fizzy drinks with far too many ingredients. Many skewing towards a candy-like sweetness, or as mundane as seltzer with tincture added. Not my desire at all! Jamie Evans has crafted a marvelously intricate book without cloying sweetness, creating some really amazing recipes that are easy to reproduce and delicious to sip.

Rather than focusing on just the history of the cannabis plant, what Jamie has achieved is a balance of her unique time-tested recipes with deeper influences that come from her years in the wine industry as a trained sommelier. Jamie's ideas for cannabis-infused cocktails are fun and easy to procure, with ingredients, unlike the ones in my own book, that are easy to prepare and to love.

What Jamie has achieved is also forthright and deeply instructional. Her book is easy to navigate, and each carefully crafted tipple offers depth and balance, which is pretty much missing from modern-day cannabis mixology. She even does a deep dive into ice (page 20). My favorite topic above all is well-made ice. Jamie takes her candid simplicity for fine ingredients and brings flavor and fragrance into the equation, making craft cocktails that are simple and fun. Her drinks are innovative classics with real aromas, timeless recipes that make the art of drinking into a perfectly memorable experience.

When you think of a perfectly crafted cannabis cocktail, your choice for humor and fancy should include the flawlessly delicious recipes that Jamie Evans has created with her attention to detail that supersedes many other drinks, both infused and uninfused, alcohol or mocktail!

I'm proud to be Jamie's friend in this "highly" competitive world of cannabis-infused libations. I may have created the science behind the art, but what Jamie has achieved makes the art of a cannabis-infused cocktail even more exciting. She has succeeded in creating an inspirational book that does more than just read well. Her drinks taste good, too!

—Warren Bobrow

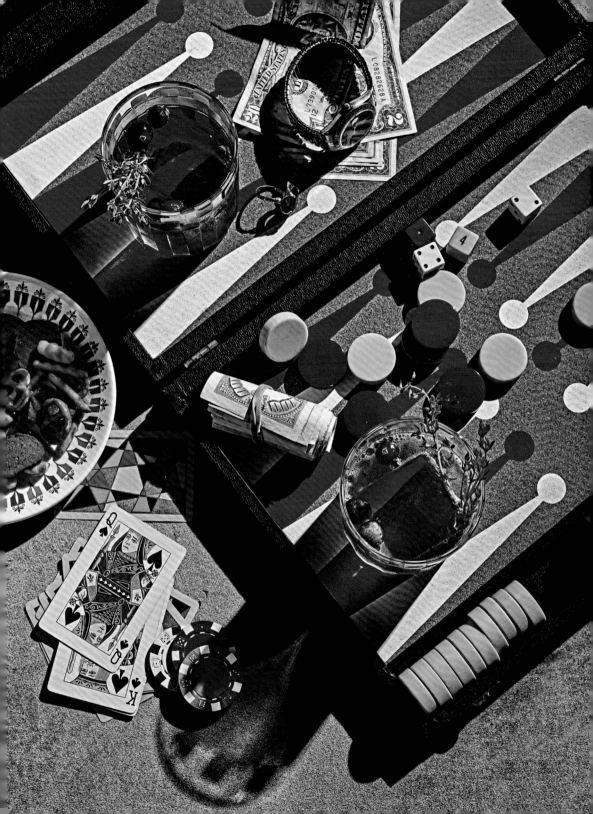

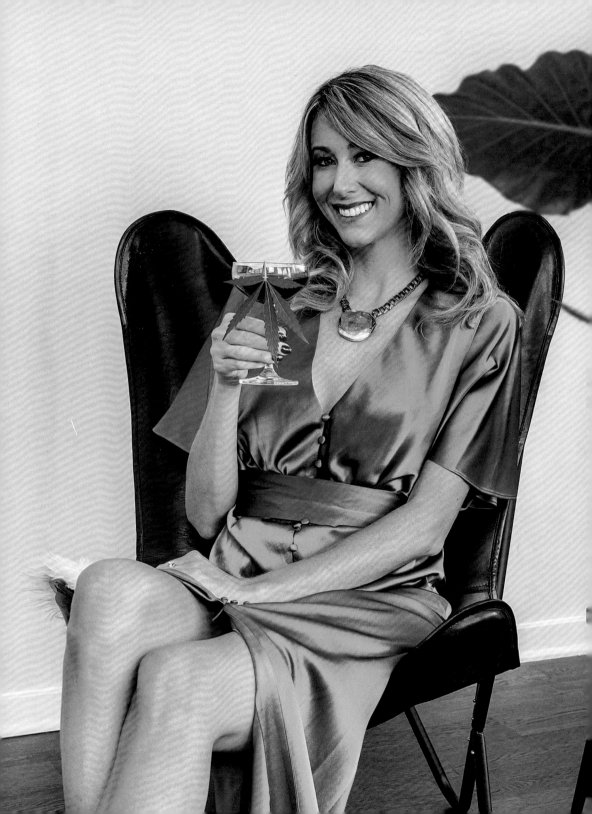

A CANNABIS DRINK
FOR EVERY OCCASION

From the time I started my career in the wine and spirits world, I've been fascinated with cannabis drinks. They capture the imagination, opening a new door to how we can enjoy our favorite beverages on an elevated level. Similar to cooking with cannabis, there's an art and science to enhancing our favorite drinkables. This begins with developing a deep understanding of and appreciation for the plant's special properties and its capacity to be used as a gourmet ingredient.

Just like the items you'd find in a thriving garden, cannabis presents a vast array of aromatic, flavorful, and therapeutic properties that masterfully intertwine with other herbs, fruits, vegetables, flowers, and spices to deliver mouthwatering flavor combinations. These flavors are especially delicious when paired with the season's freshest ingredients.

When I was approached to write a fourth book (and second book solely covering my absolute favorite category, cannabis drinks!), I knew this was the perfect opportunity to collaborate with High Times, one of the most iconic and influential cannabis platforms in the world, to bring this concept to life—a seasonal beverage book highlighting cannabis drinks for every occasion! As you work your way through this guide, the ingredients, flavor combinations, garnishes, and even drink colors are all inspired by spring, summer, autumn, and winter. These pages also honor the cannabis plant's lifecycle and growing season, as well as those who tend to these plants so dearly.

This book has been written for beginners and experts alike, so if you're here to learn more about the wonderful world of cannabis beverages, welcome home! As a Certified Sommelier and cannabis drink expert, it is my honor to guide you as we explore this delicious (and refreshing!) topic.

Before we get started, keep in mind that some of the following recipes contain alcohol. If you prefer to avoid it, you can easily adjust the recipe with the guidance provided in the "Notes" section or simply adjust it to your liking. Remember, everything in this book is customizable, so have fun with it!

Cheers to cannabis-infused beverages!

—Jamie Evans, *The Herb Somm*

CANNABIS DRINKS 101

If you're brand new to cannabis-infused drinks, this exciting category includes any beverage that's been infused with phytocannabinoids, including THC, CBD, THCV, and many others, to deliver a delightful and enhanced drinking experience. Thanks to cutting-edge technology and continued innovation, many commercially made cannabis drinks are readily available and can be enjoyed straight out of the bottle or can—infused seltzers, ciders, cannabis-infused wine, and so much more. There's something for every palate!

In addition to enjoying professionally made cannabis drinks, you can easily craft your own cannabis beverages. These drinks can deliver a buzz similar to a traditional cocktail, but crafting cannabis drinks is much different than working with alcohol because of the addition of phytocannabinoids. It's important to learn how to dose cannabis drinks *safely* and *responsibly*. We explore dosage recommendations in greater detail (page 29), but as a rule of thumb, new cannabis consumers should stay below 5 milligrams of THC per drink and consume only *one drink per session* until they're comfortable consuming more. It's also important to remember the golden rule: *Start low and go slow*—anytime you're experimenting with cannabis beverages (or with cannabis in general). Moderation is the key for an enjoyable experience!

To create the best cannabis-infused drinks possible, you can also craft your very own cannabis-infused bar pantry items (cannabis-infused simple syrups, bitters, tinctures, milk, and more). When preparing these essentials, I recommend using decarboxylated cannabis flower; however, you can also use concentrates, which tend to have more pronounced terpenes profiles (and can be less messy to work with). If you're not in the mood to make an infusion, don't worry! You can still infuse drinks by simply adding a splash of a cannabis-infused seltzer to a cocktail or adding a few drops of your favorite unflavored tincture to a smoothie or blended drink. Whatever infusion method you're most comfortable with, go for it!

> *Tip!* **Cannabis drinks are a fantastic alternative to alcohol. With new low-dose options, these beverages can offer a similar experience to drinking a glass of wine or a beer, but without any of the negative side effects. This book provides you a collection of delicious nonalcoholic cannabis-infused drinks, but it also includes a few canna-cocktail recipes that call for both cannabis and alcohol. Keep in mind that this book is customizable, so if you'd rather skip the booze, feel free to enjoy the recipe as a tasty mocktail!**

LET'S MIX IT UP!

Whether you're looking to blend up a delicious cannabis-infused smoothie or craft a cannabis cocktail, this beverage book has it all. Throughout each chapter, you learn the most practical tips and tricks to set you up for success behind the bar. In Chapter 1, you learn the basics and essentials for mixing up cannabis drinks, including how to work with cannabis flower and concentrates, techniques for pairing terpenes with seasonal ingredients, must-know mixology, and an in-depth dosage guide. Once you've learned these concepts, head to Chapter 2 for a deep dive into different infusion techniques; you'll discover how to make a series of alcohol-based infusions, fat-based infusions, and other types of cannabis infusions in the comfort of your kitchen. Finally, in Chapters 3 through 6, it's time use your new mixology skills to create cannabis drinks: seasonal smoothies, shakes, coffee drinks, juices, mocktails, and cocktails. I hope you're feeling thirsty!

> *Tip!* For readers who are already familiar with infusions and the basics of working with cannabis behind the bar, feel free to flip to Chapter 2 (page 35) to get started on the infusion recipes.

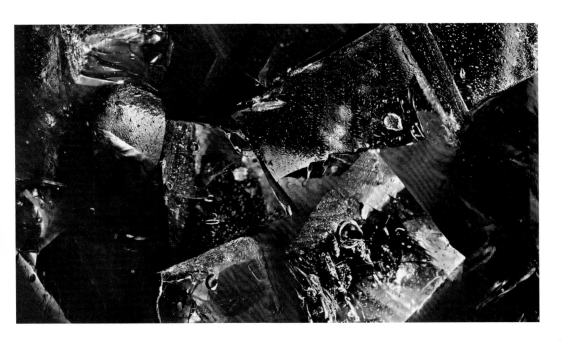

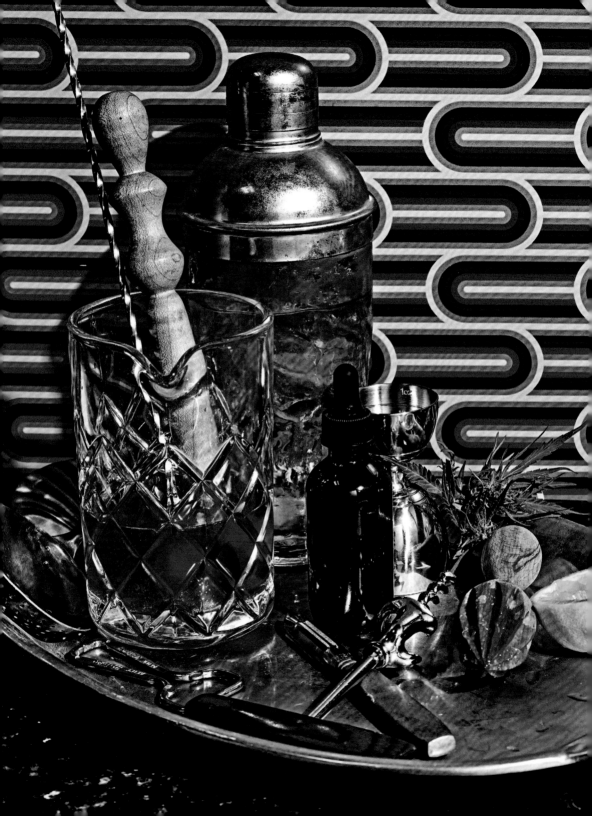

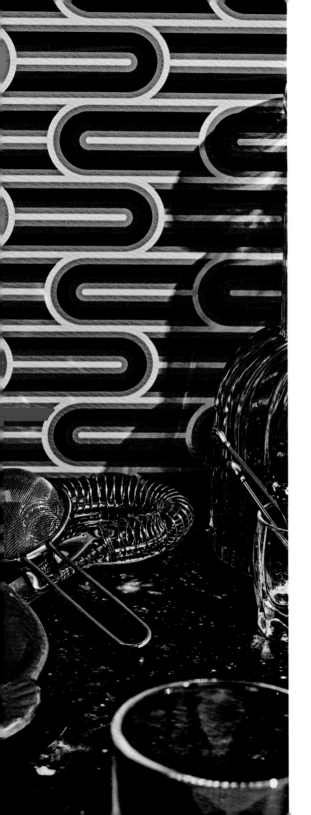

CRAFTING CANNABIS DRINKS

CHAPTER 1

If you're brand new to crafting cannabis drinks, one of the most important points to remember is that it's incredibly easy to infuse just about any beverage—there's no need to feel intimidated! With a little practice and an understanding of how the infusion process works, you will quickly become an expert at assembling deliciously infused smoothies, high teas, coffee drinks, mocktails, canna-cocktails, and more.

Throughout this chapter, we explore all these essentials, plus provide crucial mixology tips, decarboxylation info, methods for infusing drinks, instructions on dosing beverages safely and responsibly, and give you the low-down on the tools and equipment you'll need to become an expert in no time. But first, let's start with the basics.

THE BASICS

The beverage recipes found throughout this book focus on using garden-fresh, seasonal ingredients. Similar to cooking with cannabis, to craft the best-tasting cannabis-infused drinks, you'll want to source fresh cannabis items that boast an array of terpenes and phytocannabinoids to create the tastiest infusions possible. Let's take a look at two of the most popular cannabis items to infuse with: cannabis flower and concentrates.

Working with Cannabis Flower & Concentrates

In general, using cannabis flower, or hemp flower, to make infusions at home is one of the most common and approachable ways to create cannabis-infused drinks. If you're planning to source flower for your recipes, here are a few important pointers to keep in mind:

- Choose cannabis flower that best aligns with your personal needs and taste. Whether it's CBD-rich, THC-rich, or a balanced ratio (meaning cultivars that fall somewhere between CBD-rich and THC-rich, or a 1:1 ratio), use your favorite strains to craft the infusions found in this book.

- If you plan to purchase cannabis flower, always source clean, lab-tested products that are available at legal, licensed dispensaries. Be sure to look for the Certificate of Analysis (CoA), which not only highlights lab testing results, but also includes important terpene and phytocannabinoid information to help with your purchasing decision.

- Be sure to check the expiration dates on prepackaged flower. Just like with other produce, using fresh cannabis products will yield the most flavorful drink infusions.

- Choose *sun-grown* flower whenever possible, for the most unique aroma and flavor profiles. Cannabis thrives when grown outdoors under the golden sun. There's a freshness and distinctness that can be created only by the plant's sense of place, otherwise known as *terroir*. Although indoor cannabis offers some benefits, Mother Nature provides an abundance of magic that cannot be replicated.

In addition to using cannabis flower, you can infuse drinks using cannabis concentrates. As a much more potent option, concentrates are excellent for those who require a higher dose or simply want to avoid the sometimes grassy chlorophyll flavors of cannabis flower to craft infusions. Here are a few other key pointers:

- Choose *solventless* concentrates. If you're planning to use concentrates to craft your drink infusions, you'll want to use solventless concentrates, which are cannabis extracts made without the use of chemical solvents, such as CO_2 or butane. Using a solventless option ensures that your beverages will have no potentially harmful additives, which is incredibly important when ingesting cannabis. The best solventless concentrates to look for when making drinks include Ice Water Hash (or Bubble Hash), Kief, or Live Rosin (not to be confused with Live Resin, which is not solventless).

- When using concentrates to create your infusions, it's easier to estimate the total amount of THC content and dose per serving than when using cannabis flower, which can be more difficult to measure accurately. Flip to page 29 for an overview of how to calculate the dosage.

- Concentrates present more pronounced terpene notes, which adds complexity and nuance to your cannabis-infused drinks. Concentrates can also exhibit deeper earthy characteristics, which combines well with savory beverages.

- The mess is less with concentrates! When infusing with concentrates, you don't have to worry about messy flower debris during the infusion process. You'll still want to filter your infusions, but concentrates tend to yield cleaner results.

Whether you choose to use cannabis flower or concentrates to create the infusions in the next chapter, remember to have fun with it! You have so many cultivars and strain expressions to experiment with. It's always best to explore both options to determine what method works best for you.

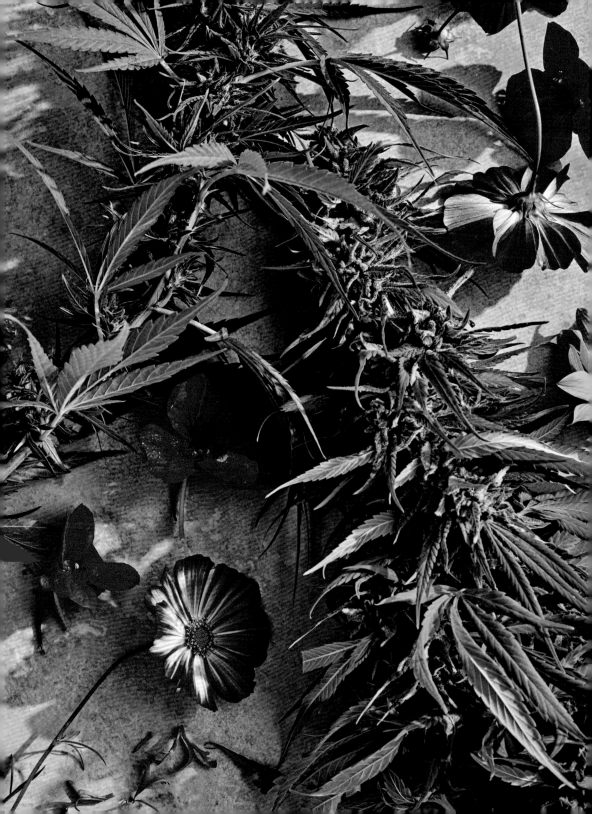

Pairing Terpenes with Seasonal Ingredients

Each season plays a critical role throughout the cannabis plant's lifecycle, from seed to harvest. Just as plants are closely connected to Mother Nature's seasonal variations, we are closely tied to the seasons as well through what we eat and drink during the year. We can celebrate seasonal ingredients from the garden and select the unique aromas and flavors of vegetables, fruits, flowers, spices, or herbs to create the most flavorful cannabis drinks.

When pairing cannabis with other ingredients, remember to lean in! As you learned at the beginning of this book, cannabis offers a broad spectrum of unique flavors and aromas, all derived from terpenes and other flavorants. We can pair cannabis with seasonal ingredients because of these special compounds. Miraculously enough, terpenes aren't found in cannabis alone—they are the building blocks of the flavors, aromas, and therapeutic properties of many different fruits, herbs, flowers, and spices that are already growing in your backyard or garden.

When crafting seasonal drinks, you'll want to highlight the smells, tastes, and colors that are reflected throughout spring, summer, autumn, and winter. Consider the following:

SPRING: Spring drinks should be fresh and vibrant, reflecting the new growth and bright flavors of the season. Think rhubarb, spring greens, carrots, roses, and sweet peas. The best cannabis terpene profiles to pair with include limonene, linalool, nerolidol, and ocimene.

SUMMER: When it comes to summer drinks, the most luscious berries, cherries, stone fruits, and tropical fruits are in season. During the warmer months, you'll want to create drinks that refresh and cool down the palate. You can best pair these drinks with cannabis strains that express higher levels of limonene, myrcene, linalool, and nerolidol.

AUTUMN: Autumnal drinks are all about celebrating spice and richness. Think cinnamon, nutmeg, cardamom, brown sugar, maple syrup, and more. One of the most flavorful holidays in the United States, Thanksgiving, is also celebrated during autumn, so adding some savory notes to a fall beverage is highly encouraged. Autumn flavors pair exceptionally well with the cannabis terpenes beta-caryophyllene and myrcene. Humulene can also present some clove, cardamom, and ginger notes, which are oh-so-perfect for fall.

WINTER: During the winter season, it's that special time of the year to mix up a variety of festive holiday drinks, but don't forget about citrus-rich beverages that boost the immune system. When it's cold outside, there's nothing more comforting than a warm beverage to keep you cozy. Winter flavors pair well with cannabis strains that exhibit pronounced levels of pinene, limonene, terpinolene, and beta-caryophyllene.

Terpene Chart

To experiment with pairing cannabis terpene profiles with your favorite seasonal ingredients, use the following terpene guide to assist you.

	BETA-CARYOPHYLLENE	HUMULENE	LIMONENE	LINALOOL
AROMAS & FLAVORS	Black pepper, cloves, cinnamon, copaiba	Hops, fresh-cut wood, coriander, cloves, cilantro, cardamom, sage, earthy notes	Lemon, lime, grapefruit, blood orange, tangerine	Lavender, citrus blossoms, citrus, violets, roses, lilies
TERPENE BENEFITS	Antianxiety, anti-inflammatory, antioxidant, pain reliever	Anti-inflammatory, antibacterial, appetite suppressant, pain reliever	Stress reliever, weight loss aid, mood enhancer	Antianxiety, sleep aid, muscle relaxant, antidepressant, antiacne
TERPENE EFFECTS	Analgesic, calm, stress free	Euphoric, relaxed, sedated	Uplifted, energized	Relaxed, blissful, rejuvenated
CANNABIS STRAINS	Omrita RX, Northern Lights, Dancehall, Rockstar	Headband, Peppermint Cookies, Gelato, GSC	Lemon Haze, OG Kush, Tangie	Pink Kush, Lavender OG, LA Confidential, Amnesia Haze

MYRCENE	NEROLIDOL	OCIMENE	PINENE	TERPINOLENE
Mixed herbs, mushrooms, forest floor, skunk, tropical fruits, mango, earthy notes	Jasmine, perfume, ginger flower, tea tree, lemongrass, floral and woody notes	Parsley, basil, mint, oregano, tarragon, bergamot, kumquat	Pine tree, pine needles, wet wood, rosemary, dill, parsley, juniper berries	Lilac, citrus, nutmeg, cumin, allspice, perfume, pine tree, sage
Sleep aid, muscle relaxant, antidepressant	Antifungal, antidepressant, sleep aid	Antioxidant, decongestant, anti-inflammatory	Asthma reliever, energy boost, anti-inflammatory	Antibacterial, antifungal, antioxidant
Sleepy, sedated	Tranquil, peaceful	Uplifted, energized	Alert, focused	Relaxed, sedated
Cannatonic, Critical Mass, Harlequin, Harle-Tsu, Pineapple Express	Island Sweet Skunk, Banana Kush, Blue Dream, Royal Cookies	Clementine, Dream Queen, Dutch Treat, Golden Pineapple	ACDC, Jack Herer, Trainwreck, Valentine X	Ghost Train Haze, Golden Goat, XJ-13, Orange Cookies

MUST-KNOW MIXOLOGY

Now that you know some of the basics, let's dive into essential mixology tips to set you up for success behind your bar. To craft the best-tasting drinks possible, a few key concepts are important to keep in mind: The first is *balance*. Whether you're working with salty, sweet, sour, bitter, or umami flavors, keeping the components balanced on your palate will guarantee a pleasurable drinking experience. When the drink is out of balance, a single ingredient might appear to be overly pronounced and create an angular effect on the palate (for example, too much sugar makes a drink taste extremely sweet, and too much acidity makes a drink taste abundantly sour). The addition of alcohol and cannabis-infused ingredients adds extra layers of flavor and complexity to the beverage. When combining these ingredients, the goal is for everything to remain balanced and to blend seamlessly together.

Achieving balance is your top priority when crafting drinks, but a few other key philosophies are necessary as you begin to master cannabis mixology. Let's begin with flavor theory.

Flavor Theory

When crafting cannabis drinks, my number one recommendation is to complement the flavors of cannabis instead of trying to mask it. This can be easily achieved by using terpene-rich ingredients such as citrus, fresh garden herbs, fruits, spices, and other ingredients to complement cannabis's natural aromas and flavors. You can also combine terpene-rich ingredients in the infusions you create (such as cannabis-infused cardamom simple syrup or mint syrup) to effortlessly blend cannabis flavors into the beverage.

When developing recipes, you'll also want to think about all the components of the drink and how their flavors and aromas might complement or contrast with each other. As with wine tasting, taste each ingredient separately and write down your tasting notes. Then continue to build the drink from there, just as a chef builds a recipe.

Exploring Ice

If you're brand new to mixing up drinks, you might be surprised to know that ice plays a *very important* role in the outcome of your beverages. Not only does ice chill a drink to refresh and awaken the palate, but cocktails and mocktails taste and look better when they're served at the correct temperature. Ice can also dilute beverages to make them more palatable (which is important for alcoholic drinks, although you never want to over-dilute your cocktails or mocktails!).

Here are some of the most common types of ice to use, along with the recommended tools and techniques for creating nice ice.

CRACKED ICE: Pieces of ice that range in size from ¼ inch to ½ inch, made from cracking ice cubes into smaller pieces. To do this at home, simply use an ice mallet or the bottom of a heavy potato masher to crack the ice cubes. Cracked ice is great for mojitos or other bubbly cocktails/mocktails.

CUBED ICE: The most common ice used, measuring around 1 inch by 1 inch. You can create these ice cubes using silicone trays. This type of ice is ideal for shaking and stirring because it doesn't dilute the drink as much as the other ice options. You can also create oversize large square ice cubes for drinks such as an old fashioned.

CRUSHED ICE: Very small pieces of ice, almost snowy (but not shaved ice like in a snow cone). This type of ice melts quickly, so it's used for only certain drinks, such as the mint julep and some tiki drinks.

Ice Tools & Equipment

The following is a quick checklist of the essential tools and equipment you'll need for all things ice.

- ☐ Ice bucket
- ☐ Ice scoop
- ☐ Ice pick and mallet
- ☐ Food-grade silicone ice mold trays with lids, including:
- ☐ Large square ice cube mold, which creates 4 to 6 large ice cubes for whiskey drinks
- ☐ Standard ice cube mold with a lid, which creates about 15 square ice cubes (best for most drinks and for creating floral ice)

Tips from the Pros:

- When creating ice cubes at home, always use filtered, clarified water (or bottled water)—not tap water! This keeps unwanted flavors out of your ice and also helps with the clarity and integrity of your drinks.

- Most often, the ice in your freezer is not the best choice for cocktails or mocktails, but it will do just fine in a blended drink, if ice is necessary.

- When working with crushed ice, never add it to your cocktail shaker! The tiny ice pieces will melt and greatly dilute your drinks.

- When making ice cubes using silicone trays, use hot water. The water will freeze slowly, creating crystal-clear ice cubes. Cold water produces unwanted air bubbles, which can cloud the ice.

- When making drinks, shake or stir the beverage for 15 to 30 seconds to achieve the best temperature and dilution for a cocktail before straining it into a glass. For mocktails, shake or stir for 15 seconds or until cold without overdiluting. Pay close attention to the directions in each recipe found in this book for specific chilling times.

How to Make Floral Ice

When you're in the mood to be creative and take your drinks to the next level, you can create floral ice cubes, in which a cannabis leaf or edible flower is frozen into the middle of the ice cube. To prepare floral ice at home, use a standard silicone ice cube mold. Choose the edible flower or leaf of your choice (preferably cannabis leaves, if you can access them). Place the flowers or leaves into the silicone ice tray, spreading them out evenly. Fill each ice cube mold halfway with hot filtered or bottled water (not tap water!). Don't fill the ice cubes all the way just yet; if you do, the flowers or leaves will float to the top, creating an uneven appearance. Place the trays into the freezer, and chill until frozen. Remove the ice tray, and then top each ice cube again with warm filtered water so that the rest of the ice cube fills out. Place the tray into the freezer, and chill overnight. When the ice is frozen, use your floral ice cubes in any drink that needs a boost of color and festive flair!

Mixing Techniques

Depending on how you craft your cannabis beverages, the infused ingredients will either blend gracefully with your other liquid ingredients or separate (like oil and vinegar). As a budding cannabis mixologist, you do not want separation to occur! Your goal is to keep the liquid as homogenous as possible, so that the drink is accurately dosed and your phytocannabinoids and other precious cannabis compounds don't get stuck to the bottom or sides of the glass. With this is mind, it's typically not recommended to use oil-based tinctures (or CBD oil) in drinks because of their affinity to separate; the exception is if you're preparing a blended recipe—then the blender will emulsify all of your ingredients together without encountering loss.

Using a blender works wonders for combining cannabis into drinks, but it's not the only technique you can use to emulsify cannabis into a beverage. Another common strategy is shaking. To shake a drink properly, using a shaker tin or Boston shaker is recommended; if you don't currently own this equipment, a mason jar with a sealable lid works just as well. Simply add the ingredients into the shaker, shake well to combine, and then strain the emulsified liquid into the recommended glassware. As a rule of thumb, any beverage that calls for citrus, fresh fruit juices, egg whites, or dairy (or other "cloudy" ingredients) should be shaken. When you shake, the added oxygen helps boost the flavors of these ingredients, or it creates a creamy mouthfeel.

> *Note:* **Don't add anything carbonated to your shaker tin. It will explode, and you'll have a big mess to clean up.**

In addition to blending and shaking, you can use a muddler to combine cannabis infusions into your beverages (hello, canna-mojitos!), or use a mixing glass and a bar spoon to vigorously stir everything together. Throughout this book, you will use all these strategies to craft cannabis drinks, along with a few other clever methods to enhance your beverages (such as a cannabis-infused salted rim!).

How to Safely Mix Cannabis & Alcohol

As you're working through the next chapters, you'll come across recipes that call for both cannabis *and* alcohol. When it comes to mixing the two together, moderation is the key to an enjoyable experience. To avoid feeling dizzy and sick, always keep safe and responsible consumption in mind. When creating cannabis-infused alcohol cocktails, I recommend staying below 10 milligrams of THC per drink (or between 1 and 2.5 milligrams of THC, if you're a beginner). Start low, go slow, and remember to be patient! It can take up to an hour or more to feel the effects of cannabis, so do not consume more than one drink unless you are very experienced at consuming both alcohol and cannabis at the same time and you know your limits. You should also *never* mix cannabis-infused cocktails with other medications and *never* drive or operate machinery after consuming. Remember to drink responsibly!

In addition to mixing cannabis with alcohol in a canna-cocktail, you'll be using alcohol to extract phytocannabinoids when crafting some of the infusions in the next chapter (i.e., for tinctures and bitters). As you will discover, ethanol is a potent solvent that allows you to successfully capture these precious cannabis compounds while blending harmoniously into other liquids. When mixing with an alcohol-based infusion, you'll use only a small portion to infuse a drink, so you won't experience any effects from the alcohol after it's consumed (unless additional alcohol is called for the recipe). Flip to page 39 for an alcohol-based infusion recipe.

> *Note:* **Mixing cannabis and alcohol might not be for everyone. Keep in mind that you can always skip the booze in the canna-cocktail recipes and choose to make an alcohol-free version instead.**

CANNABIS COOKING ESSENTIALS

Now that you're familiar with some cannabis basics and mixology principles, let's dive into a few cannabis cooking essentials. In this section, you learn how to properly decarboxylate cannabis, explore different methods for infusing beverages, discover how to safely dose drinks, calculate the dosage per serving, and find a list of all the equipment and tools you'll need to craft the recipes.

DECARBOXYLATION

To create the most successful cannabis infusions, you must decarboxylate your cannabis before you integrate it into a recipe. If you're new to decarboxylation, this is a heating process that triggers a chemical reaction, releasing the carboxylic acids from CBD and THC to fully activate the cannabis (that is, you are converting THCA to THC and CBDA to CBD).

Many approaches to decarboxylation are practiced, including using the oven, a device, or the sous vide to decarb. The most common method, known as the oven method, exposes cannabis to heat at 240°F to 295°F (115°C to 146°C) for 20 to 60 minutes. Heat for a shorter time at higher temperatures, or for a longer time at lower temperatures.

To decarboxylate at home, the following are some simple heating instructions for both cannabis flower and concentrates using the oven method.

To Decarboxylate Flower

Preheat your oven to 240°F (115°C). As your oven is heating up, line a baking sheet with parchment paper or aluminum foil. While wearing gloves, use your fingers (or scissors) to break up the cannabis flower into pea-size pieces, and spread them evenly onto the baking sheet. When the oven is heated, simply put the baking sheet in the oven and bake for 20 to 30 minutes. Remove from heat, let cool, and store in an airtight sealed mason jar until you're ready to use.

To Decarboxylate Concentrates

Preheat your oven to 200°F to 240°F (93°C to 115°C). Remember, lower temperatures are better for concentrates. As the oven preheats, transfer the concentrate into a small oven-safe clear glass baking dish (or any clear dish allows you to keep an eye on the heating process). Cover the baking dish with a lid or aluminum foil to prevent excess evaporation, and then place the dish into the oven. Once your concentrate has completely liquified and is consistent, it's decarboxylated. You can also use a thermometer to check the internal temperature to verify this.

> *Note:* When using the oven to decarb, be aware that your kitchen will fill up with *very potent* cannabis aromas during the heating process. If you live in a building where your neighbors or landlord might take notice, it's best to use a decarboxylation or sous vide device to decarb your weed, to best conceal the aromatics (see "Resources," on page 148, for my favorite recommended devices).

Activation Temperatures for Decarboxylation

Stay within these temperature ranges to properly decarboxylate your cannabis. Be mindful not to exceed 300°F (150°C) at any time because you'll diminish the precious phytocannabinoids and terpenes that you're trying to preserve.

Phytocannabinoids	°F	°C
THCA*	240–275	115–135
CBDA**	240–295	115–146

*Converts from THCA to THC if you heat between 240°F and 275°F (115°C and 135°C) for 20 minutes to 1 hour
**Converts from CBDA to CBD if you heat between 240°F and 295°F (115°C and 146°C) for 20 minutes to 1 hour
***Sourced from *Cannabis Drinks: Secrets to Crafting CBD and THC Beverages at Home*

METHODS FOR INFUSING DRINKS

As you will learn throughout this book, there are many ways to infuse your favorite beverages. If creating homemade infusions isn't your thing, don't worry! You can enhance your drinks in several other easy ways. Here's an overview of the primary methods.

Infusions

When crafting cannabis drinks, the best way to enhance a beverage is to create an infusion. Making an infusion is a process of extracting compounds (such as THC and CBD) from cannabis using a solvent such as an alcohol- or fat-based solution (such as oil or butter). By allowing the cannabis to be suspended in the solvent over time, the cannabis compounds bind with the fats and alcohol to create a cannabis-infused substance. Although alcohol and fat tend to be the best solvents for extraction, other considerations can do the job, depending on what you're creating. Let's quickly explore all these options.

ALCOHOL-BASED INFUSIONS: In the following pages, you learn how to craft two primary alcohol-based infusions for drinks: bitters and tinctures. Ethanol (also known as grain alcohol) is the source of extraction for this method and yields potent results when combined with cannabis. When working with alcohol-based infusions, these can be created either at room temperature or with low heat to best extract cannabis compounds. If you decide to use heat, take extra precautions! Heating can speed up the infusion process, but it can be dangerous: Alcohol is *extremely flammable* and has a low boiling point—always keep temperatures far below 170°F (77°C). For these reasons, I recommend using only the sous vide to heat these infusions. Never use the gas stove or an open flame.

FAT-BASED INFUSIONS: When preparing beverages that call for some cannabis-infused cream (or butter), you'll want to create a fat-based infusion. Because phytocannabinoids and other cannabis compounds are naturally drawn to fats and are fat soluble, these special molecules easily bind with fat-based liquids, creating an enhanced ingredient to mix with. For the purposes of this book, you will learn how to create cannabis-infused butter, milk, and cream, along with super creamy coconut milk. If you don't consume dairy milk products, you can easily swap for soy milk or hemp milk.

OTHER CONSIDERATIONS: From time to time, you might come across an infusion that doesn't call for a fat- or alcohol-based ingredient. In these instances, you might use vegetable glycerin (mostly for syrups and simple syrup), honey, or maple syrup. Although these ingredients typically do not yield as potent results as alcohol or fat, they still extract cannabinoids and can serve as a sufficient infusion to sweeten your drinks. In Chapter 2, you learn how to work with these considerations to build out your cannabis bar pantry.

COMMERCIALLY MADE PRODUCTS

If cooking isn't your thing, you'll be overjoyed to learn that a variety of commercially made products can easily enhance just about any recipe. From prepacked cannabis-infused seltzers to cannabis-infused sugar, these gourmet products are designed to make your life easy. One of the greatest benefits of using a commercially made product is that it is precisely dosed. Due to stringent cannabis laws and regulations, any product that you find at a legal, licensed dispensary is required to list the dose per serving on the product packaging so you will know exactly how much THC you've consumed. On the other hand, it's very difficult to determine the exact dosage of homemade infusions, so it's essential to calculate an estimate based on the source material you're using. That said, if you prefer an easier route to infusing beverages, using a commercially made product might be your preferred method.

TINCTURES: Using a commercially made tincture to infuse a beverage is a quick and beginner-friendly way to enhance beverages. Although oil-based tinctures tend to separate from other liquid ingredients, you can still successfully incorporate them into shakes, smoothies, and blended mocktails or cocktails using a blender to powerfully emulsify all your ingredients together. Tinctures also enable you to easily titrate your dose up or down until you find your perfect ratio, making this method a great option for those who are brand new to mixing drinks with cannabis. If you're planning to use a tincture, make sure that it's *unflavored*, to avoid any unwanted aroma and flavor additions to your beverages. In this book, you learn how to create an alcohol-based tincture; flip to page 42 for the recipe.

> *Note:* **Depending on the tinctures you have at home and your taste preferences, you could follow the lead of some mixologists and add a few drops of CBD or THC oil to float on the top of the drink, to add a pleasant complexity and a silky, round mouthfeel to certain drinks. If the tincture is terpene forward, it can also add a boost of aromatics. (Just don't be surprised if you find some oil stuck to the bottom or side of your glass after consuming it, which isn't ideal)**

OTHER PANTRY ITEMS: Here are a few other commercially made cannabis-infused products to look for: honey, sugar, sriracha, hot sauce, olive oil, apple cider vinegar, chili oil, cannabis-infused drink mixers, and powdered mixers. Flip to "Resources," on page 148, for a listing of my favorite items available at this time of writing this book.

A QUICK GUIDE TO DOSING

Whether you're preparing a cannabis cocktail or making your favorite cannabis-infused cuisine, ensuring safe and responsible dosing is crucial, especially when working with THC and its derivatives. Determining the exact dosage per serving in homemade drinkables and edibles can be difficult—you'll never be 100 percent accurate because many factors can influence the outcome, including ingredients used, evaporation, heating methods, and cannabinoid loss due decarboxylation/cooking. Knowing this, always follow the golden rule: *Start low and go slow.*

For the purposes of this book, the recipes included fall between 5 and 10 milligrams THC per serving. If you're brand new to cannabis, stay between the range of 1 to 5 milligrams, for best results. For cannabis aficionados, feel free to increase the dosage to best suit your needs. For those who solely want CBD, stay between 5 and 25 milligrams of CBD per drink (even though consuming a blend of phytocannabinoids is recommended).

The Dosage Calculation

The cannabis infusions highlighted in these pages were crafted from a selection of cannabis flower measuring at a total of 15 percent THC and 1 percent CBD before decarboxylation. In each recipe, you'll see a target dose listed based on these numbers, to use as a baseline; however, the potency of your infusions will differ, depending on the strain and source of the product you use. With this in mind, always be sure to calculate your own THC/CBD milligrams per serving to best gauge the potency.

> *Note:* **The potency of your infusions will most likely be a little lower than your estimated dosage per serving because of cannabinoid loss during decarboxylation and a loss of volume due to evaporation during the infusion process. Knowing this, it's crucial to sample ⅛ to ¼ teaspoon (or whatever amount you're comfortable with) to test the potency on yourself before serving to others.**

The following page illustrates a step-by-step formula to calculate the dosage per serving (adapted from the book *The Ultimate Guide to CBD,* Fair Winds Press, 2020). After you've done the math, always use measuring spoons, droppers, and cups to dose as accurately as possible.

STEP 1: Convert the THC and CBD percentages to determine the milligrams per gram of dry flower (1 gram = 1,000 milligrams). The total amount of THC and CBD in your product should be listed on the packaging when you purchase it.
Example: Based on the values for Vanilla Frosting, 15% THC and 1% CBD
    0.15 x 1,000 mg/g = 150 mg THC per gram of dry cannabis flower
    0.01 x 1,000 mg/g = 10 mg CBD per gram of dry cannabis flower

STEP 2: Multiply the mg/g of THC and CBD from step 1 by the grams of flower called for in your recipe.
Example: For coconut milk, a recipe calls for 3.5 grams of cannabis flower.
    150 mg/g x 3.5 grams = 525 mg THC
    10 mg/g x 3.5 grams = 35 mg CBD

STEP 3: Convert your primary infusion ingredients (coconut milk, butter, milk, high-proof grain alcohol, and so on) into grams.
Example: 3 cups coconut milk = 750 grams

STEP 4: Calculate the number of servings remaining in your final yield. Divide your answer from step 3 by the number of grams per serving indicated in the following chart.
Example: 750 grams of coconut milk ÷ 28.5 grams of coconut milk per ounce = About 26 ounces of coconut milk

Ingredient	Serving size	Grams
Butter	1 tablespoon	14.18
Milk	1 ounce	28
Coconut milk	1 ounce	28.5
Simple syrup	1 ounce	28
Alcohol bitters and tinctures	1 milliliter	0.789

STEP 5: Divide your THC and CBD amounts from step 2 by the number of servings in step 4 to calculate the THC and CBD per serving.
Example: Final calculation for coconut milk
    525 mg ÷ 26 ounces = About 20 mg THC per ounce, or about 10 mg THC per half-ounce
    35 mg ÷ 26 ounces = About 1.35 mg CBD per ounce, or about < 1 mg CBD per half-ounce

Essential Tools & Equipment

As you work your way through each recipe, you'll notice that specific equipment is listed. These tools will help you create the beverage as recommended, but you don't need to purchase all the items. Feel free to improvise with the tools you already own (check your inventory). Here's a list of recommended tools and equipment to best set you up for success behind the bar:

- ☐ Amber glass bottles with dropper caps
- ☐ Bar spoon
- ☐ Blender or food processor
- ☐ Candy or instant-read thermometer
- ☐ Cheesecloth
- ☐ Citrus press
- ☐ Digital scale
- ☐ Double jigger
- ☐ Fine-mesh strainer
- ☐ Funnel
- ☐ Glass syrup bottle with stainless steel pourer
- ☐ Hawthorne strainer

- ☐ Mason jars, varying sizes
- ☐ Measuring glass (1 to 5 ounces)
- ☐ Mixing glass
- ☐ Muddler
- ☐ Oven mitt
- ☐ Peeler
- ☐ Saucepans, varying sizes
- ☐ Shaker tin
- ☐ Sous vide precision cooker
- ☐ Spice grinder
- ☐ Vacuum seal
- ☐ Vacuum seal bags
- ☐ Whisk

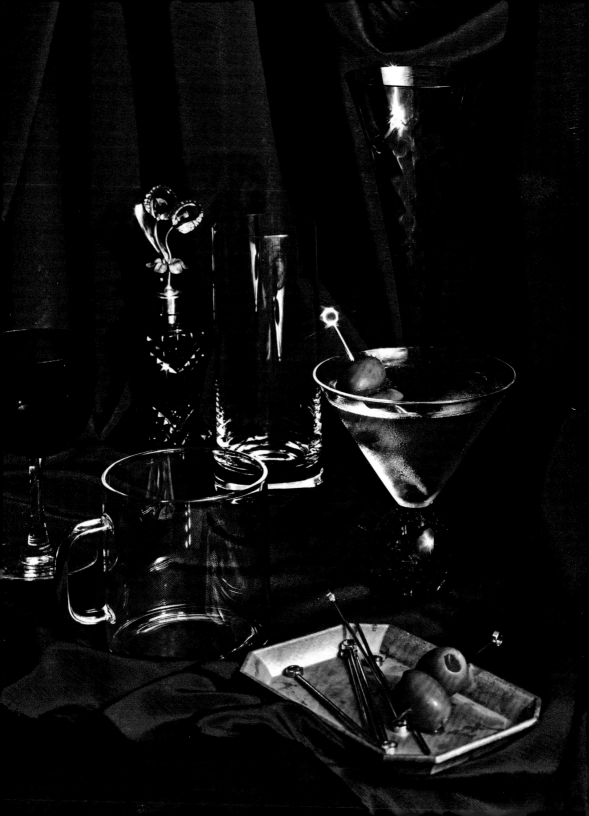

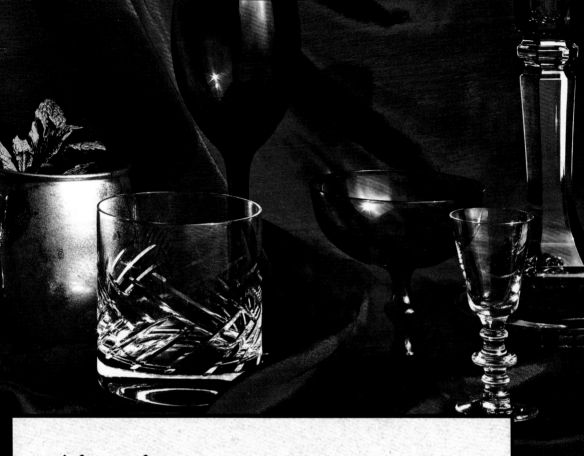

A Guide to Glassware

Choosing the appropriate glassware for serving your beverages is an essential part of crafting the most flavorful drinks. Depending on what you're mixing up behind the bar, certain glasses pair best with certain cocktails, mocktails, juices, smoothies, and more. Here are a few highlighted glasses to have on hand when working with this book:

- ☐ Classic mug
- ☐ Copper mug
- ☐ Coupe glass
- ☐ Highball glass
- ☐ Old fashioned glass/rocks glass

- ☐ Shot glass
- ☐ Sour glass
- ☐ Stemless wine glass
- ☐ Wine glass

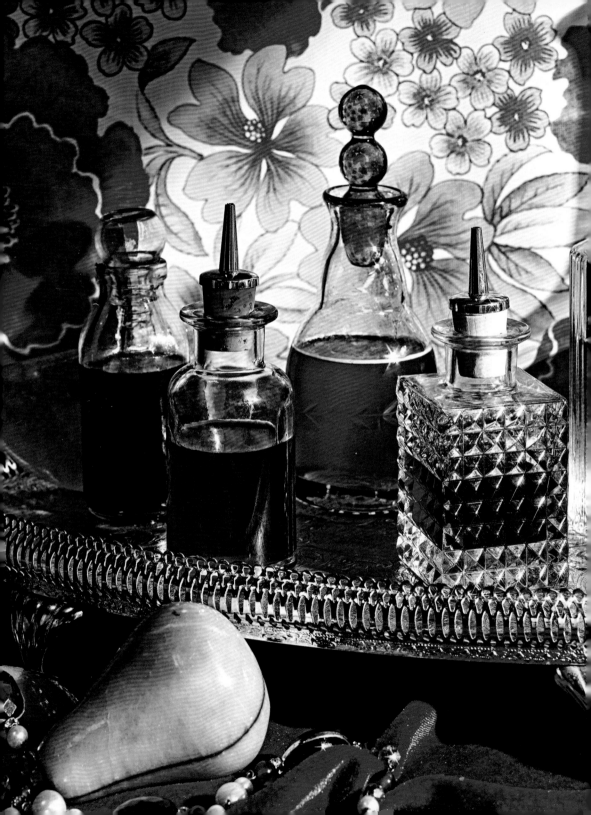

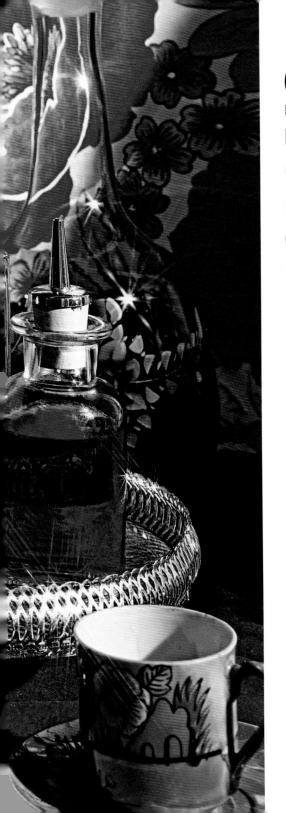

CRAFTING INFUSIONS

CHAPTER 2

There's no better way to elevate a beverage than to create a cannabis infusion. Whether you're using an alcohol- or fat-based solvent or some other type, you can easily craft a variety of homemade infusions that will add unique aromas, flavors, complexity, depth, and phytocannabinoids to your favorite drinks. Now that you have an understanding of the basics of cannabis drinks and cooking essentials, it's time to use what you've learned and start mixing!

This chapter features all the cannabis infusions that you'll need to elevate the drinks throughout this book. Before you reach the recipes, this chapter also includes the most common methods used to create infusions—you have the option to choose what method works best for you.

THE INFUSION GUIDE

When creating infusions at home, you will use several different methods to best extract phytocannabinoids from the cannabis ingredients you're working with. Fat-based infusions require heat to begin the infusion process, but when preparing alcohol-based infusions, you can extract at freezing temperatures, room temperature, or low-heated temperatures— it all depends on what infusion you're creating. Let's explore the three most common methods for preparing infusions, which are also the methods highlighted in this book.

Tip! If you don't have the time to create these infusions, or if cooking isn't your thing, rest assured that all the drink recipes found in this book can also be enhanced using your favorite *unflavored* THC or CBD tincture (an alcohol-based tincture is best) or a commercially made pantry item. If you decide to go this route, simply swap the infused item that's called for in the recipe for the noninfused version (such as swapping Cannabis-Infused Maple Syrup for plain maple syrup), and then proceed with the recipe as directed using a tincture or commercially made item. Keep an eye on the "Note" section at the bottom of each recipe for the directions.

3 Methods for Preparing Infusions

To craft the infusions found in this chapter, you can choose to use the stovetop method, the sous vide method, or, for alcohol-based infusions, the old-school mason jar method to extract cannabis compounds into a number of bar pantry items. The following is a quick overview of each method before we get to the recipes.

The Stovetop Method

The stovetop method is one of the most common and approachable ways for preparing infusions at home. Using the equipment you most likely already own, including a stove (or heat plate), a small saucepan, a thermometer, a cheesecloth, and a fine-mesh strainer, you can heat fat-based ingredients or other liquids (besides alcohol) over heat for an extended period of time to extract phytocannabinoids and other cannabis compounds. For best results, I recommend staying between 160°F and 180°F (71°C and 82°C) when heating; be careful not to exceed 200°F (93°C), to prevent your infusion from getting close to boiling! When using this method, keep a close eye on your infusion, to protect it from overheating, and continue to stir from time to time, to assist with an even extraction.

The Sous Vide Method

If you already own a sous vide device, the sous vide method might be your infusion method of choice. Using the sous vide offers many benefits: It keeps your infusion at a constant temperature, and you can "set and forget" without having to keep a constant eye on the infusion process, as when using the stovetop method. You can also heat alcohol-based infusions using the sous vide, as long as you keep temperatures far below 170°F (77°C)— alcohol is flammable at this point. For best results, I recommend heating alcohol-based infusions at 140°F (60°C) for 2 hours. For fat-based infusions, you can heat for longer at higher temperatures, but keep in mind that lower temperatures are always preferable, to protect the integrity of your phytocannabinoids and terpenes.

The Old-School Mason Jar Method

The final method of infusion highlighted in this book is the old-school mason jar method. You'll want to use this easy method when crafting alcohol-based infusions (and if you don't already own a sous vide device). For this technique, all you need is a high-proof grain alcohol (preferably, 80 proof or higher), your cannabis base ingredient (cannabis flower or concentrates), and a mason jar. Simply add the ingredients to the jar, shake to combine, and then store in a dark pantry or the freezer for the amount of time directed. For the best extraction, you'll want to shake daily to best capture the cannabis compounds. This method takes several days to extract cannabis compounds, but it's reliable and safe because you're not exposing alcohol to heat. This method is primarily used to craft bitters and tinctures.

INFUSION RECIPES

This section includes the infusion recipes used to craft the drinks in this book. These recipes were crafted using cannabis flower, which measured at a total of 15 percent THC and 1 percent CBD before decarboxylation. Remember, the target dosages included in each recipe can be used as a baseline for your infusions, but depending on what flower, concentrate, or other cannabis product you're using, your final outcome will vary. Flip to page 30 to calculate the estimated milligrams per serving, to ensure safe and responsible dosing.

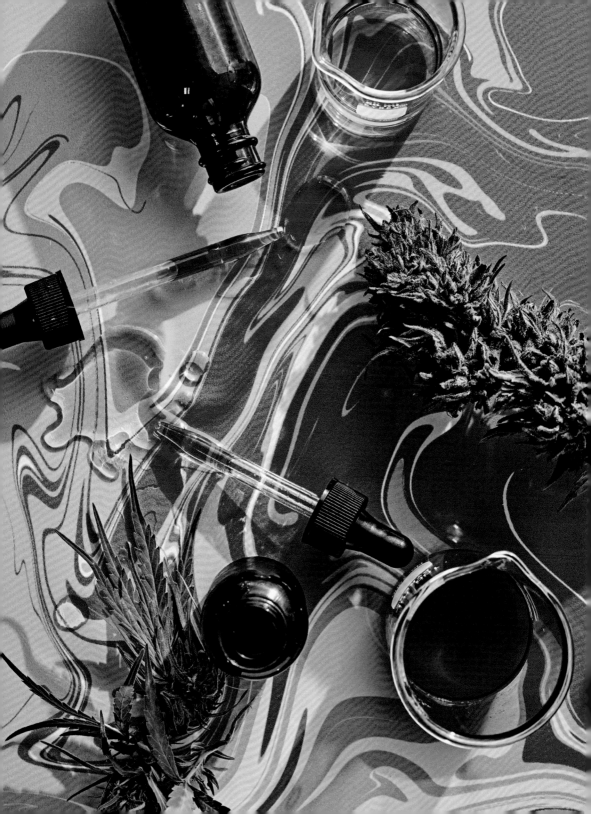

CANNABIS-INFUSED BUTTER

Whether you're cooking or mixing up cannabis drinks, infused butter adds a creamy texture and buttery flavors to hot drinks, making them oh-so-comforting and delicious. You can also use Cannabis-Infused Butter to fat-wash alcohol, which makes spirits a bit smoother and creamier.

TARGET DOSE:

9 mg THC | 1 mg CBD per teaspoon

28 mg THC | 2 mg CBD per tablespoon

*These numbers will differ, depending on the strain and source of the product you use.

EQUIPMENT:

Digital scale

16-ounce (480 mL) sterilized tempered glass mason jar

Measuring cup

Medium saucepan

Thermometer

Oven mitt

Cheesecloth

Fine-mesh strainer

Silicone butter stick tray or the storage container of your choice

INGREDIENTS:

3 to 4 grams decarboxylated cannabis flower of your choice (use 4 grams for a stronger dose)

1 cup (227 g) unsalted European butter (with a minimum of 82% milk fat)

1. Weigh out the decarboxylated cannabis flower of your choice.

2. Cut the butter into cubes, and then combine in a tempered glass mason jar with the cannabis flower. Be sure to put the butter on the bottom of the jar so it melts properly. Seal the top tightly.

3. In a medium saucepan, fill the bottom of the pan with water, allowing enough space so that the water will not hit the top of the mason jar. Set the mason jar inside, and begin to heat on low. Continue to heat to just below 200°F (93°C) for 2 hours, making sure the water does not exceed 211°F (99°C). Check in frequently, and refill the pan with water as needed due to evaporation. Agitate the jar every now and then using an oven mitt. When finished, remove the mason jar safely with an oven mitt, and let the jar cool.

4. Prepare the cheesecloth by placing it over the fine-mesh strainer. Pour the infused butter over the cheesecloth into a clean measuring cup or mason jar to remove the solids and flower debris. Gently press to extract the butter, but don't squeeze the cheesecloth: This will extract bitter chlorophyll notes and green color! Filter a few times as needed.

5. Once filtered, pour the clarified butter into a silicone butter stick mold tray, and cover. Put in the refrigerator overnight so that it resolidifies and hardens. The next day, use a knife to loosen the sides of the infused butter sticks, and drain out any liquid that might have separated out at the bottom of the tray.

6. To store, wrap each butter stick separately in plastic wrap, label the sticks, and keep chilled in the refrigerator. To freeze for use later, wrap each stick with plastic wrap and then aluminum foil, for extra protection.

CANNABIS-INFUSED MILK

Cannabis-Infused Milk is especially delicious in coffee or tea drinks, providing a tasty, creamy enhancement! When preparing this recipe at home, keep in mind that milk and milk substitutes tend to evaporate quickly on the stovetop. Keep a very close eye on the heat, and continue stirring to break up any film that may form at the top of the liquid during the infusion process. During the fall and winter seasons, you can also add some spices, such as cinnamon and nutmeg, to create spiced milk (or cream). If stored in the refrigerator in an airtight bottle or container, this recipe should stay fresh for up to two weeks.

TARGET DOSE:

5 to 6 mg THC | < 1 mg CBD per half-ounce

10 to 11 mg THC | 1 mg CBD per ounce

*These numbers will differ, depending on the strain and source of the product you use. Be sure to factor in 12.5% loss of liquid due to evaporation.

EQUIPMENT:

Scale

Measuring cups

Measuring spoons

Small saucepan

Thermometer

Cheesecloth

Fine-mesh strainer

24-ounce (710 mL) mason jar

INGREDIENTS:

1.5 to 3 grams decarboxylated flower of your choice (use 3 grams for a stronger dose, but it will taste and look greener)

3 cups (720 mL) whole milk (or substitute cream, coconut milk, soy milk, or hemp milk)

½ teaspoon vanilla extract

1. Weigh out the decarboxylated flower of your choice. Set aside.

2. Combine the milk and vanilla extract in a saucepan, and then begin to heat on low. Add the cannabis, and continue to heat until it reaches 160°F to 180°F (71°C to 82°C). Keep a close eye on the infusion: Be careful not to overheat and boil the milk!

3. As the milk continues to infuse, stir frequently to break up the film on top, and scrape the sides to remove any deposits.

4. After 1 hour of cooking, remove the infused milk from heat. Some of the milk will evaporate, so you will have less than your original 3 cups.

5. Using a fine-mesh strainer and cheesecloth, strain the infused milk into an airtight container or mason jar for storage.

6. Let cool, and then put in the fridge to chill before serving. If you don't want to use dairy milk, you can use coconut milk, soy milk, or hemp milk for this infusion. You can also use cream, which will happily bind with your cannabis compounds.

> *Note:* **To prepare this recipe using the sous vide, simply set your sous vide bath to 160°F (71°C). Combine the decarboxylated cannabis flower with the milk of your choice in a tempered glass mason jar (seal tight!) or sous vide pouch. Place into the sous vide bath, and heat for 1 hour. Then follow the previous directions.**

FAT-BASED INFUSIONS

CANNABIS-INFUSED SUPER CREAMY COCONUT MILK

This rich infusion is creamier than traditional coconut milk, which makes it ideal for blended drinks and smoothies. It's also ideal for capturing phytocannabinoids because of the added coconut fat. To infuse at home, using the sous vide method is recommended, to prevent evaporation (see note), but you can also prepare this recipe on the stovetop. During the infusion process, keep a close eye on the coconut milk to make sure it doesn't boil.

TARGET DOSE:

5 to 6 mg THC | < 1 mg CBD per half-ounce

10 to 11 mg THC | 1 mg CBD per ounce

*These numbers will differ, depending on the strain and source of the product you use. Be sure to factor in 35% to 40% loss of liquid due to evaporation.

EQUIPMENT:

Digital scale

Measuring cups

Small saucepan

Thermometer

Silicone spatula

Cheesecloth

Fine-mesh strainer

Airtight storage container of your choice

INGREDIENTS:

1 to 3 grams decarboxylated flower of your choice (use 3 grams for a stronger dose, but it will taste and look greener)

2 cups (480 mL) coconut milk

⅓ cup unsweetened coconut cream (see "Resources," on page 148)

1. Weigh out the decarboxylated flower; set aside.

2. Add the coconut milk and coconut cream to a saucepan over medium heat. Heat to 160°F to 180°F (71°C to 82°C), and then add the decarboxylated cannabis.

3. Keep a close eye on the temperature, stirring frequently and scraping the sides of the saucepan to remove any flower debris and to break up the film.

4. After 50 minutes of cooking, remove the infused coconut milk from heat. Line a fine-mesh strainer with cheesecloth, and then pour the coconut milk through to filter out any flower debris.

5. Strain again, if needed; then transfer the infused coconut milk into an airtight container of your choice for storage. A portion of the milk will evaporate, so you will have less than your original amount of coconut milk. Transfer the infused coconut milk into the container of your choice, let cool, then store in the refrigerator until further use. This recipe should stay fresh for up to 2 weeks.

Tip! **For this recipe, you'll want to use coconut milk that's meant to be refrigerated and that won't solidify when chilled.**

Note: **To avoid evaporation, use a sous vide and set your sous vide bath to 160°F (71°C). Combine the decarboxylated cannabis flower with the coconut milk and unsweetened coconut cream in a tempered glass mason jar (seal tight!) or vacuum-sealed sous vide pouch. Place into the sous vide bath, and heat for 1 to 2 hours. Then follow the previous directions.**

FAT-BASED INFUSIONS

THE CLASSIC CANNABIS-INFUSED TINCTURE, THREE WAYS

As one of the most versatile bar pantry items, learning how to craft an alcohol-based tincture to infuse your drinks is indispensable. Not only will this infusion blend seamlessly with your other liquid ingredients, but tinctures are a key component to other pantry items you'll create in this book, including cannabis-infused grenadine, coffee syrup, salt, and sugar. If you decide to use the heated method to prepare the tincture, keep in mind that it will have a much darker color and stronger cannabis notes, compared to the freezer method (which is not as clean looking/tasting because heat accelerates the extraction of everything, including chlorophyll). However, this process produces faster and more potent results if you're in need of a quick infusion.

TARGET DOSE:

4 mg THC | < 1 mg CBD per milliliter

113 mg THC | 10 CBD per ounce

*These numbers will differ, depending on the strain and source of the product you use.

EQUIPMENT:

16-ounce (480 mL) mason jar

Fine-mesh strainer

Cheesecloth

Airtight storage container of your choice, or split between amber glass bottles with dropper caps

INGREDIENTS:

7 grams decarboxylated flower of your choice

1 cup (240 mL) high-proof clear grain alcohol (120 proof or higher)

1. Combine 7 grams of decarboxylated flower with 1 cup (240 mL) high-proof clear grain alcohol in a mason jar. Seal the jar tightly, and place it in the freezer for 10 days. Shake the jar every day to help with the extraction process.

2. After the 10 days, line a fine-mesh strainer with cheesecloth, and filter out the solids from the infused alcohol.

3. Store in an airtight container of your choice or in amber glass bottles with dropper caps. For best results, filter a few times to help with clarity. Store in the refrigerator for several months.

Sous Vide Tincture

If you currently own a sous vide, you can create this infusion in 2 hours versus 10 days! Remember, the sous vide is the safest heating method to use when preparing this recipe; you should never heat alcohol over a gas stove or open flame.

1. To prepare at home, set your sous vide bath to 140°F (60°C).

2. Combine 1 cup high-proof clear grain alcohol with 7 grams of decarboxylated cannabis into a tempered glass mason jar (seal tight!) or an airtight vacuum-seal pouch made for sous vide.

3. Place the jar or pouch into the sous vide bath, and heat for 2 hours.

4. Using an oven mitt or tongs, remove from heat; let cool to room temperature.

5. Line a fine-mesh strainer with cheesecloth, and strain into an airtight container of your choice or amber glass bottles with dropper caps. For the best clarity, filter a few times to remove all flower debris. Store in the refrigerator for several months.

Fresh Flower Tincture

1. Combine 7 grams of fresh flower (not decarboxylated) with 1 cup (240 mL) high-proof clear grain alcohol in a mason jar. Seal the jar tightly, and place it in the freezer for 10 days. Shake the jar every day to help with the extraction process.

2. After the 10 days, line a fine-mesh strainer with cheesecloth, and filter out the solids from the infused alcohol.

3. Store in an airtight container of your choice or in amber glass bottles with dropper caps. For best results, filter a few times to help with clarity. Store in the refrigerator for several months.

> *Tip!* **Fresh flower tinctures are fantastic for showcasing the cannabis plant's unique terpene profile because the alcohol extracts these aromatic and flavorful compounds without encountering loss from heat. You'll also be able to harness the benefits of the nonintoxicating phytocannabinoids THCA and CBDA if the flower isn't decarboxylated, so it's a great alternative, depending on your needs.**

CANNABIS-INFUSED CARDAMOM CINNAMON BITTERS

In the cocktail world, bitters are used as a flavoring agent to help blend drink flavors. Made from different bittering ingredients (cinchona bark, horehound, and so on) sourced from bark, roots, or dried herbs, these special alcohol-based elixirs are combined with fruits, flowers, spices, and other natural ingredients (including cannabis!) to create flavorful combinations that enhance just about any mixed beverage.

TARGET DOSE:

3 mg THC | < 1 mg CBD per ¼ teaspoon, or 2 dashes (12 to 16 drops)

74 mg THC | 5 mg CBD per ounce

*These numbers will differ, depending on the strain and source of the product you use.

EQUIPMENT:

One 32-ounce (940 mL) sterilized mason jar

Two 16-ounce (480 mL) sterilized mason jars

One 8-ounce (240 mL) sterilized mason jar

Cheesecloth

Fine-mesh strainer

Airtight swing bottle or amber bottle with a dropper cap

INGREDIENTS:

10 grams decarboxylated flower of your choice

10 cardamom pods, cracked

1 cinnamon stick

4 whole dried allspice berries

¼ cup dried orange peels

1 tablespoon dried sour cherries

1 (1-inch) piece fresh ginger, peeled and sliced into pieces

½ teaspoon cinchona bark

2 cups (480 mL) high-proof rye (80 proof or higher)

Add if diluting (see instructions right):

¾ cup water

½ ounce noninfused simple syrup (optional)

1. Using a 32-ounce mason jar, add the decarboxylated cannabis flower, cracked cardamom pods, cinnamon stick, allspice berries, dried orange peels, dried sour cherries, ginger, and cinchona bark to the bottom of the jar.

2. Top with high-proof rye, seal with an airtight lid, and shake vigorously. Make sure all your ingredients are fully submerged into the rye.

3. Steep this mixture for 10 days, stored in a dark cabinet. Be sure to shake daily for the best extraction.

4. When the 10 days are up, separate the solids from the liquids over a clean 16-ounce (480 mL) mason jar using a fine-mesh strainer and cheesecloth. Seal the mason jar filled with the filtered infused bitters, and store it in a dark cabinet until further use. If you want stronger-tasting and more potent bitters, follow the steps as directed, but infuse for 2 weeks or more.

> *Tip!* To increase the shelf life of your bitters, store them in an amber glass bottle instead of clear glassware. However, you'll want to use clear glassware during the infusion process so you can keep an eye on the color and ingredients.

To dilute the bitters (if using a high-proof spirit [120 proof or more])

1. Follow the previous steps. Then after filtering, transfer the solids into a saucepan, and top with ¾ cup (175 mL) water. Begin to heat over medium heat for 5 to 6 minutes.

2. Remove from heat, and let cool. When the mixture reaches room temperature, transfer it to a clean 16-ounce (480 mL) mason jar, and steep for 3 days in the refrigerator, shaking daily.

3. When the 3 days are up, separate the liquid from the solids using a fine-mesh strainer and cheesecloth into a clean 8-ounce (240 mL) mason jar; discard the solids/sediment. For the best clarity, filter a few times to remove all leftover debris. Add this liquid mixture to the infused rye that you've already created, and then add the simple syrup (if using).

4. Shake well. Let the bitters rest for a few additional days, allowing any leftover sediment to sink to the bottom of the mason jar.

5. When ready, carefully filter out the clean liquid resting on top using a fine-mesh strainer and cheesecloth. Leave the sediment behind; then discard.

6. To best preserve your bitters, transfer the liquid into dark glassware or amber glass bottles. Store at room temperature in a dark cabinet for several months.

The Heated Sous Vide Method

If you own a sous vide device, follow this recipe for the fastest and safest way to create this type of infusion with heat.

1. To prepare at home, set your sous vide bath to 140°F (60°C). Combine the decarboxylated cannabis flower, cracked cardamom pods, cinnamon stick, allspice berries, dried orange peels, dried sour cherries, ginger, cinchona bark, and high-proof rye in a tempered glass mason jar (seal tight!) or an airtight vacuum-seal pouch made for sous vide.

2. Place the pouch or jar into the sous vide bath, and heat for 2 hours. Using an oven mitt or tongs, remove from heat; then let cool to room temperature.

3. Separate the solids from the liquids over a clean 16-ounce (480 mL) mason jar using a fine-mesh strainer and cheesecloth.

4. Seal the mason jar filled with the filtered infused rye, and store it in a dark cabinet until further use.

5. To dilute, follow the previous instructions.

BACON FAT-WASHED MEZCAL

If you're new to fat-washing, this is an extraction method that occurs between fat flavor compounds and alcohol. Spirits such as mezcal are best for this method because they have the ability to extract and dissolve fatty flavors into the liquid, leaving behind a decadent fat-flavored spirit. When using a cannabis-infused fat (in this case, bacon fat), this process allows cannabis compounds to be extracted and infused into the alcohol (at 80 proof or higher) that you're working with, creating a delicious, smooth, and creamy alcohol base for cannabis cocktails.

TARGET DOSE:

6 to 7 mg THC | < 1 mg CBD per ½ ounce

13 to 14 mg THC | < 1 mg CBD per ounce

*These numbers will differ, depending on the strain and source of the product you use. Because this infusion is combined with alcohol and intended to be used in a cocktail, it's best to stay below 10 mg THC per ½ ounce so you don't overdo it.

INGREDIENTS:

3.5 grams decarboxylated flower of your choice

¾ cup (180 mL) bacon fat

¼ cup (60 mL) liquified cannabis-infused bacon fat

2 cups (480 mL) mezcal

EQUIPMENT:

Digital scale

8-ounce (240 mL) sterilized mason jar

Saucepan

Thermometer

Fine-mesh strainer

Cheesecloth

32-ounce (940 mL) sterilized mason jar

16-ounce (480 mL) sterilized mason jar or airtight swing-top bottle

1. Weigh out 3.5 grams of decarboxylated cannabis flower.

2. In a mason jar, combine the cannabis flower and bacon fat. Seal the top tightly. If you're using a bacon fat that's hardened, be sure to melt it down to measure exactly ¾ cup (180 mL).

3. In a small saucepan, fill the bottom of the pan with water, making sure to allow enough space so that the water will not hit the top of the mason jar. Set the mason jar inside (seal it tight!), and begin to heat until the water reaches 180°F to 200°F (82°C to 93°C). Heat for 2 hours, making sure the water does not exceed 211°F (99°C).

4. Check in frequently, and refill the pan with water as needed, due to evaporation.

5. When finished, safely remove the mason jar with an oven mitt, and let the jar cool.

6. Prepare the cheesecloth by placing it over the fine-mesh strainer. Pour the infused bacon fat over the cheesecloth into a clean mason jar, and then set aside to cool (but not harden!).

7. When the cannabis-infused bacon fat has cooled, measure out ¼ cup. In a 32-ounce (940 mL) sterilized mason jar, add the mezcal and cannabis-infused bacon fat. Top with a lid, and then vigorously shake the two ingredients together.

8. Place the mason jar in the freezer for 24 hours (or until the fat solidifies at the top of the mason jar).

9. Remove from the freezer, poke a hole through the side of the solidified bacon grease, and then strain the liquid through a fine-mesh strainer lined with cheesecloth to catch any leftover solids and debris. Repeat until the liquid contains no solids.

10. Transfer to a clean 16-ounce (480 mL) sterilized mason jar or airtight swing-top bottle, and store in the refrigerator for up to 2 weeks. You might need to filter again as the fat particles resolidify.

Tip! **To collect the greatest amount of bacon grease possible for this fat-wash, place the raw bacon strips on top of a warmed nonstick sauté pan. Begin to heat until the bacon becomes crispy; then drain the grease into an 8-ounce mason jar. Be sure to run the grease through a fine-mesh strainer, to remove any bacon pieces. It might take a few pounds of bacon to yield ¾ cup, depending on the type of bacon you use, so be sure to purchase at least two 2-pound packages when preparing this recipe. Enjoy the bacon and save the grease to infuse with cannabis as directed!**

CANNABIS-INFUSED HONEY

Whether you're adding it to a beverage or eating it with a spoon, Cannabis-Infused Honey is one of the most scrumptious items you'll have in your pantry. Drizzle canna-honey on top of your favorite desserts, or easily combine it into smoothies, hot drinks, and more! If you're in a rush and you don't have the time to infuse the honey on your stovetop, you can also blend honey with your favorite tincture to infuse (see note). If you use this method for infusion, be sure to use measuring spoons to precisely dose.

TARGET DOSE:

9 mg THC | 3 mg CBD per teaspoon

28 mg THC | 8 mg CBD per tablespoon

*These numbers will differ, depending on the strain and source of the product you use.

EQUIPMENT:

Digital scale

Small saucepan

Silicone spatula

Cheesecloth

Fine-mesh strainer

Tempered glass container with lid

Thermometer

INGREDIENTS:

3 grams decarboxylated flower of your choice

1 cup (340 g) honey

2 teaspoons food-grade vegetable glycerin

1. Weigh out the decarboxylated cannabis.

2. In a small saucepan, using a thermometer, heat the honey to 170°F (77°C). Stir in the cannabis and vegetable glycerin.

3. Simmer over low heat for 1 hour, constantly stirring and checking the temperature.

4. Line a fine-mesh strainer with cheesecloth, and pour the infused honey into the tempered glass jar with a lid.

5. Before each use, give the honey a big stir if any separation occurs from the vegetable glycerin. Use within 3 weeks for the best flavor.

> *Note:* If you don't have the time to infuse the honey on the stovetop, add 1½ teaspoons (or your desired amount) of tincture and 1 cup honey to a blender. Blend on high speed for a couple minutes, and then empty the infused honey into a mason jar. Let your infused honey settle, and give it a good stir before serving. If separation occurs over time, re-emulsify by blending the honey again.

CANNABIS-INFUSED SIMPLE SYRUP

This classic recipe can be made using a variety of sugar bases, which deliver different flavor profiles to your beverages. Simple syrups made from granulated sugar tend to be the most neutral, and simple syrups using agave nectar, honey, or brown sugar can add more depth and a richer flavor. You'll use several different simple syrups throughout this book, so be sure to bookmark this recipe.

TARGET DOSE:

8 to 9 mg THC | < 1 mg CBD per half-ounce

16 to 17 mg THC | 1 to 2 mg CBD per ounce

*These numbers will differ, depending on the strain and source of the product you use.

EQUIPMENT:

Digital scale

Saucepan

Silicone spatula

Measuring cups

Thermometer

Cheesecloth

Fine-mesh strainer

Airtight storage container of your choice

INGREDIENTS:

2.5 to 4 grams decarboxylated flower of your choice (use 4 grams for a stronger dose, but it will taste greener)

2 cups (480 mL) water

3 cups (600 grams) granulated sugar (or brown sugar)

2 tablespoons food-grade vegetable glycerin

1. Weigh out the decarboxylated cannabis, and set aside.

2. Add the water and sugar base of your choice to a small saucepan over medium heat. Stir until the sugar base dissolves completely into the water.

3. Reduce the heat to 160°F to 180°F (71°C to 82°C). Add the decarboxylated cannabis and vegetable glycerin and stir to combine.

4. Simmer over low heat for 1 hour, occasionally stirring, scraping the sides of the pan to remove flower debris. Remove from heat.

5. Line a fine-mesh strainer with cheesecloth, and pour the infused simple syrup into the container of your choice to separate out the solids. For the best clarity, filter the simple syrup a few times through the cheesecloth to catch all leftover debris. Let cool; store in the refrigerator until further use. Always shake before serving.

How to Make Cannabis-Infused Honey Simple Syrup

1. Weigh out 2 grams of decarboxylated cannabis, and set aside.

2. Add 2 cups (480 mL) water and 1¼ cup (425 g) honey to a small saucepan over medium heat. Stir until the honey dissolves completely into the water.

3. Reduce the heat to 160°F to 180°F (71°C to 82°C). Add the decarboxylated cannabis and 1 tablespoon vegetable glycerin and stir to combine.

4. Simmer over low heat for 1 hour, occasionally stirring, scraping the sides of the pan to remove flower debris. Remove from heat.

5. Line a fine-mesh strainer with cheesecloth, and pour the infused simple syrup into the container of your choice to separate out the solids. For the best clarity, filter the simple syrup a few times through the cheesecloth to catch all leftover debris. Let cool; then store in the refrigerator until further use. Always shake before serving.

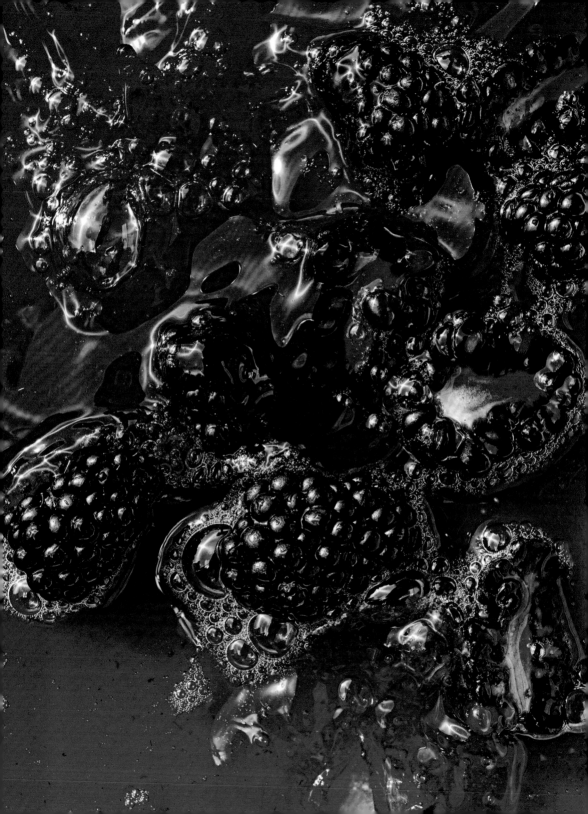

CANNABIS-INFUSED BLACKBERRY SIMPLE SYRUP

This easy-to-make recipe is similar to creating simple syrup, but you'll be extracting the flavor (and color) of fresh blackberries before infusing the syrup with cannabis. Although this recipe calls for blackberries, you can easily swap for raspberries or strawberries.

TARGET DOSE:

7 to 8 mg THC | < 1 mg CBD per half-ounce

14 to 15 mg THC | 1 mg CBD per ounce

*These numbers will differ, depending on the strain and source of the product you use. Be sure to factor in 20% to 25% loss of liquid due to evaporation.

EQUIPMENT:

Digital scale

Saucepan

Silicone spatula

Potato masher or fork

Measuring cups

Cheesecloth

Fine-mesh strainer

Thermometer

Airtight storage container of your choice

INGREDIENTS:

2.5 to 3.5 grams decarboxylated flower of your choice (use 3.5 grams for a stronger dose, but it will taste greener)

2½ cups (600 mL) water

2½ cups (500 grams) granulated sugar

2½ cups fresh blackberries

1½ tablespoons food-grade vegetable glycerin

1. Weigh out the decarboxylated cannabis, and set aside.

2. In a small saucepan, bring the water and sugar to a soft boil, stirring occasionally until the sugar dissolves.

3. Remove from heat, and stir in the blackberries. When the blackberries have warmed up, use a fork or potato masher to mash the berries into a pulp.

4. Cover the saucepan, and steep for 1 hour. Strain through a fine-mesh strainer lined with cheesecloth.

5. Transfer the fruit syrup to a clean saucepan, and heat to 160°F to 180°F (71°C to 82°C). Add the decarboxylated cannabis and vegetable glycerin; stir to combine.

6. Simmer over low heat for 1 hour, occasionally stirring, scraping the sides of the pan to remove flower debris. Remove from heat.

7. Line a fine-mesh strainer with cheesecloth; then pour the infused fruit simple syrup into the container of your choice to separate out the solids. For the best clarity, filter the syrup a few times through the cheesecloth to catch all leftover debris.

8. Let cool, and store in the refrigerator until further use. Use within 2 weeks, and always shake before serving.

CANNABIS-INFUSED COFFEE SYRUP

Calling all coffee lovers! This Cannabis-Infused Coffee Syrup is the perfect addition to warm coffee drinks and cold brew. Drizzle it on ice cream, add it to your favorite iced coffee (see page 86), combine it into an espresso martini, and so much more! Made with the strongest coffee you have access to, this syrup provides a boost of energy while keeping those coffee jitters at bay due to the addition of cannabis. For best results, use your Cannabis-Infused Tincture from page 42.

TARGET DOSE:

4 to 4.5 mg THC | < 1 mg CBD per half-ounce

8 to 9 mg THC | < 1 to 1 mg CBD per ounce

*Using the Cannabis-Infused Tincture on page 42. These numbers will differ, depending on the strain and source of the product you use.

EQUIPMENT:

Saucepan

Silicone spatula

Measuring cups

Whisk

Airtight storage container of your choice

INGREDIENTS:

1½ cups (300 grams) granulated sugar

1 cup (240 mL) strong brewed coffee (see note)

1 ounce (30 mL) Cannabis-Infused Tincture (see page 42)

I. In a small saucepan, heat the sugar and coffee over medium heat, stirring occasionally until the sugar dissolves.

2. When the sugar has fully melted into the coffee, remove from heat.

3. Let cool to room temperature; then whisk in the Cannabis-Infused Tincture. Stir well to combine.

4. Transfer into an airtight bottle or mason jar, and store in the refrigerator until further use. This infusion should last for up to a month, if stored properly. Remember to always shake well before using.

> *Note:* **To make strong coffee, brew 1½ cups water with 3 tablespoons of dark ground French roast, and then follow the directions as noted. See "Resources," on page 148, for the coffee I use, but also feel free to use your favorite brand!**

CANNABIS-INFUSED SALT

If you're a fan of salted cocktail rims, this recipe was made for you! Combining fine-grain sea salt with your Cannabis-Infused Tincture on page 42, this easy-to-make recipe will playfully enhance any drink when you're craving a sweet/salty combination (who's ready for a cannabis margarita?). When preparing at home, keep the salt exposed to open air, to allow the alcohol to fully evaporate and the salt to recrystallize. Oil-based tinctures don't work for this recipe, so be sure to use the Cannabis-Infused Tincture on page 42 for best results.

TARGET DOSE:

4 to 5 mg THC | < 1 mg CBD per teaspoon

226 mg THC | 20 mg CBD per cup

* Using the Cannabis-Infused Tincture on page 42. These numbers will differ, depending on the strain and source of the product you use.

EQUIPMENT:

Digital scale

Measuring cups

Parchment paper

Glass bowl or glass baking dish (the more surface room to spread out the salt, the faster it will dry)

Cheesecloth

Silicone spatula

Airtight glass container

INGREDIENTS:

2 cups (400 grams) fine-grain sea salt

4 ounces (120 mL) Cannabis-Infused Tincture (see page 42)

1. Pour the salt into a clear glass baking dish, followed by the Cannabis-Infused Tincture on page 42. Stir well with a silicone spatula, making sure all the salt granules are thoroughly coated in the tincture.

2. Make sure it is evenly spread for drying.

3. Cover the baking dish with cheesecloth, and secure the top with a rubber band or string.

4. The most important step in this infusion process involves airflow: Don't cover the dish with a lid. Place in a dry, unbothered area where this mixture can air-dry for about 2 to 3 days. Be sure to stir every day, to help the alcohol evaporate more quickly and to allow for an even infusion.

5. Depending on the humidity and weather in your region, the timing may vary. When all the moisture from the alcohol has completely evaporated and the consistency is similar to the kind of salt you started with, it's done! Store in a dry, airtight container, and be sure to use measuring spoons to measure the dosage as accurately as possible.

OTHER INFUSIONS

CANNABIS-INFUSED MAPLE SYRUP

Cannabis-Infused Maple Syrup? Yes, please! This easy-to-make recipe is a fantastic addition to breakfast, brunch, and a variety of mixed drinks. When choosing a maple syrup to infuse with, opt for 100 percent pure maple syrup instead of fake maple syrup that's been made with high-fructose corn syrup—ick! Be sure to read the label. Pure maple syrup has a much better flavor and isn't sticky and cloying like the artificial options.

TARGET DOSE:

8 mg THC | 3 mg CBD per half-ounce

16 mg THC | 5 mg CBD per ounce

*These numbers will differ, depending on the strain and source of the product you use. Be sure to factor in 10% to 12.5% loss due to evaporation.

EQUIPMENT:

Digital scale

Saucepan

Silicone spatula

Cheesecloth

Fine-mesh strainer

Glass container with lid

Thermometer

INGREDIENTS:

1.5 to 3.5 grams decarboxylated flower of your choice (use 3.5 grams for a stronger dose, but it will taste greener)

2 cups (480 mL) maple syrup

1 tablespoon food-grade vegetable glycerin

1. Weigh out the decarboxylated cannabis.

2. In a saucepan, using a thermometer, heat the maple syrup to 160°F to 180°F (71°C to 82°C); stir in the cannabis and vegetable glycerin.

3. Heat over low heat for 1 hour, constantly stirring, scraping the sides of the pan, and checking the temperature.

4. When finished, line a fine-mesh strainer with cheesecloth. Pour the infused maple syrup into a glass jar with a lid, back into the maple syrup container, or into an airtight bottle of your choice.

5. Before each use, be sure to give the maple syrup a shake or stir, to re-emulsify the ingredients in case any separation occurs.

> *Note:* This recipe can also be prepared using your sous vide device, which will help prevent evaporation. Simply set your sour vide to 170°F (77°C). As the water bath is heating, combine the decarboxylated cannabis with the maple syrup and vegetable glycerin. Heat for 1 hour, and then follow the directions as noted.

CANNABIS-INFUSED SUGAR

As a perfect addition to mojitos, coffee, or other beverages that need a touch of sweetness, Cannabis-Infused Sugar is a versatile ingredient that you'll want to line your pantry with. For powdered sugar, simply follow the recipe as directed, but once the Cannabis-Infused Sugar has recrystallized, grind the granulated sugar into a fine powder using a mortar and pestle. Your infused powdered sugar can then be combined with other colorful powders to create stencil artwork on top of foamy drinks such as a latte or a sour.

TARGET DOSE:

3 to 4 mg THC | < 1 mg CBD per teaspoon

226 mg THC | 20 mg CBD total

* Using the Cannabis-Infused Tincture on page 42. These numbers will differ, depending on the strain and source of the product you use.

EQUIPMENT:

Measuring cups

Parchment paper

Glass bowl or glass baking dish (the more surface room to spread out the sugar, the faster it will dry)

Cheesecloth

Silicone spatula

Airtight glass container

INGREDIENTS:

1¼ cups (250 grams) granulated sugar

2 ounces (60 mL) Cannabis-Infused Tincture (see page 42)

1. Pour the sugar into a clear glass baking dish, followed by the Cannabis-Infused Tincture. Stir well with a silicone spatula, making sure all the sugar granules are thoroughly coated in the tincture. Make sure it is evenly spread for drying.

2. Cover the baking dish with cheesecloth, and secure the top with a rubber band or string.

3. As with your salt infusion, the most important step in this process is exposing the sugar to open air. Don't cover the dish with a lid, or the alcohol will not evaporate.

4. Place in a dry, unbothered area where this mixture can air-dry for about 2 to 3 days. Be sure to stir every day, to help the alcohol evaporate more quickly and to allow for an even infusion.

5. When all the moisture from the alcohol has completely evaporated and the consistency is similar to the kind of sugar you started with, this recipe is ready! Store in a dry, airtight container, and be sure to use measuring spoons to measure the dosage per serving as accurately as possible.

> *Tip!* When the alcohol has fully evaporated from the sugar, the sugar may harden and form clumps if you don't consistently stir it every day as it's drying. Don't fret! Simply break apart the clumps by using a mortar and pestle to grind the sugar into small particles again. You'll also want to use a fork to break up any clumps that form while storing.

CANNABIS-INFUSED GRENADINE SYRUP

If you're looking to enhance your cannabis bar party, there's nothing quite like homemade grenadine syrup. Made with pomegranate juice, granulated sugar, and a touch of lemon juice, this mouthwatering recipe tastes so much better than store-bought grenadine. Plus, it's infused with cannabis to heighten cocktail hour. For best results, use your Cannabis-Infused Tincture on page 42 to infuse this recipe.

TARGET DOSE:

2.5 to 3 mg THC | < 1 mg CBD per half-ounce

5 to 6 mg THC | < 1 mg CBD per ounce

*Using the Cannabis-Infused Tincture on page 42. These numbers will differ, depending on the strain and source of the product you use.

EQUIPMENT:

Saucepan

Silicone spatula

Measuring cups

Whisk

Airtight storage container of your choice

INGREDIENTS:

1½ cups (360 mL) pomegranate juice

1½ cups (300 grams) granulated sugar

¾ ounce (22 mL) freshly squeezed lemon juice, pulp removed

1 ounce (30 mL) Cannabis-Infused Tincture (see page 42)

1. In a small saucepan, combine the pomegranate juice and sugar. Begin to heat over medium heat, stirring occasionally, until the sugar fully dissolves.

2. Add the lemon juice, and stir to combine; then remove from heat.

3. Let cool to room temperature, and whisk in the Cannabis-Infused Tincture. Whisk well to combine.

4. Transfer into an airtight bottle or mason jar, and store in the refrigerator until further use. This infusion should last up to a month, if stored properly. Remember to always shake well before using.

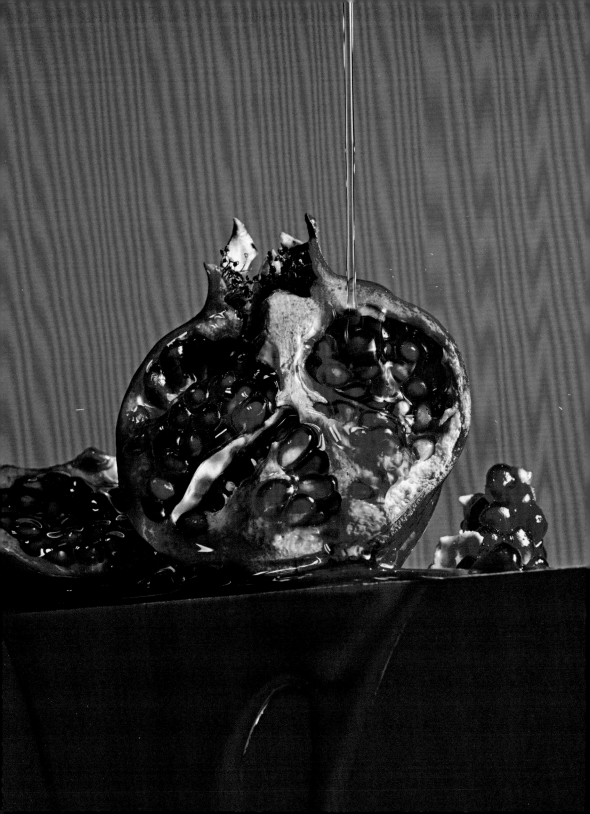

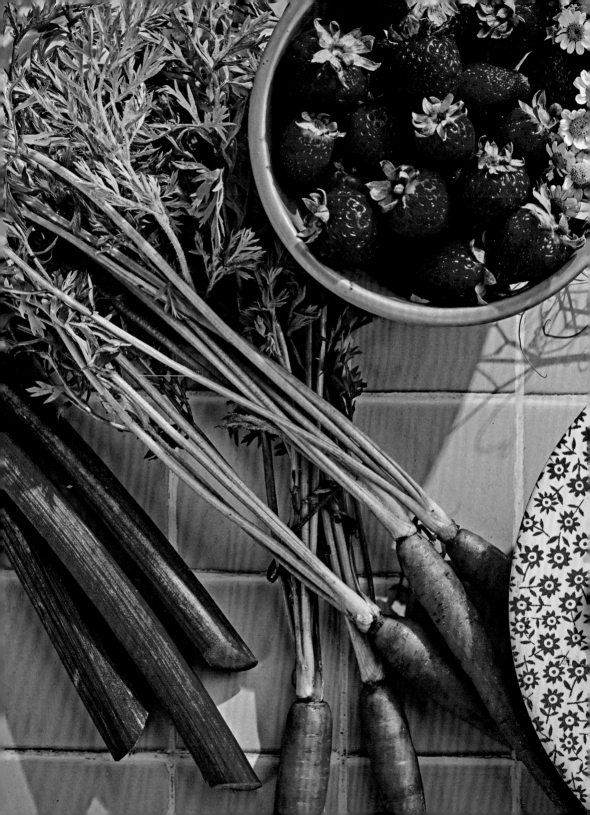

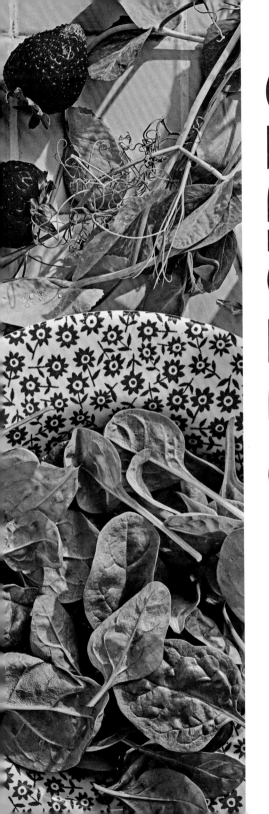

SPRING RECIPES

CHAPTER 3

Spring is that special time of year when we celebrate new life and the start of the growing season. Fresh herbs, flowers, and other botanicals are in bloom, providing a vast array of flavorful ingredients to mix drinks with. This is also the time when new seeds are planted, rooting deep into the earth to yield a bountiful crop at harvest. In this chapter, you discover recipes that incorporate these fresh, new, and vibrant flavors and pair perfectly with cannabis. From juices to smoothies, mixed drinks, and more, prepare your palate for all things spring!

SPRING GREENS JUICE

Bright, tart, and delicious, nothing says spring like a spring greens juice! This nutrient-packed recipe celebrates everything green and is the perfect kickstart when you're craving something healthy in the morning. The best way to access cannabis leaves is to grow your own plants (even though your plants will be smaller during this time of year). By juicing fresh cannabis leaves, you'll be able to access nonintoxicating THCA and CBDA, which is one of the best ways to harness the benefits of these phytocannabinoids. If you don't quite have 2 handfuls of cannabis leaves, you can either mix them with kale or use kale as a substitute.

TARGET DOSE:

Nonintoxicating THCA and CBDA

EQUIPMENT:

Juicer

Glass of your choice

INGREDIENTS:

2 handfuls fresh cannabis leaves (or 3 to 4 full kale leaves)

1 handful fresh spinach leaves

½ chilled English cucumber, cut in half

1 chilled lime, cut into quarters and peeled

¼ cup fresh mint leaves

1 chilled large green apple, cut into slices (or whatever variety of apple you prefer)

1. Feed the cannabis leaves (or kale), spinach, cucumber, lime, mint, and apple into a juicer, alternating the ingredients as you continue to juice.

2. When everything is juiced, stir to combine.

3. Pour the juice into a serving glass of your choice, and enjoy immediately. This recipe should yield around 13 ounces (390 mL) of fresh green juice.

> *Note:* Although the apple provides some sweetness to this green juice, if you'd like to add more, simply drizzle some honey into the juice after juicing, or add a few slices of pineapple to the juicer (even though it's not green) and follow the recipe as directed.

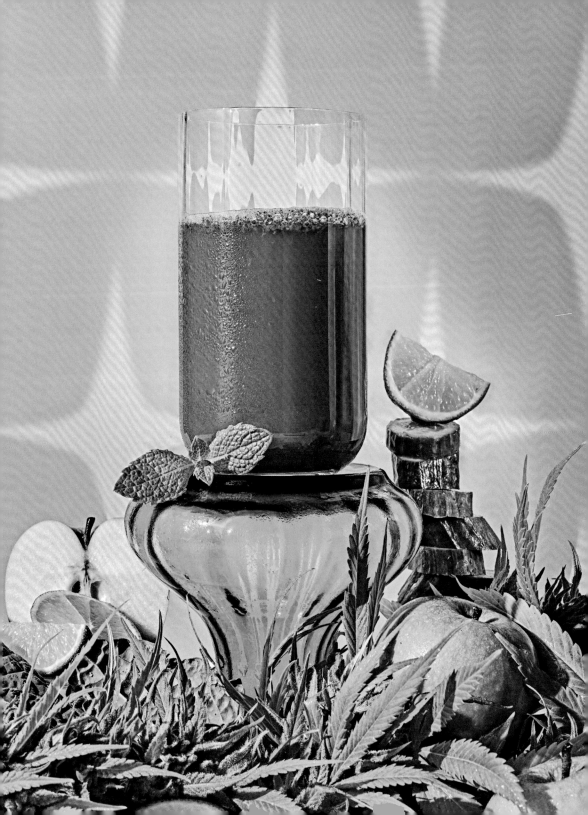

LAVENDER HAZE LATTE

Tapping into the healing powers of the terpene linalool (which is abundant in lavender and many other calming flowers and botanicals, including cannabis), nothing is more comforting than a Lavender Haze Latte. Bonus points if you've infused the milk using the Lavender Haze cannabis strain!

TARGET DOSE:

5 to 6 mg THC | < 1 mg CBD per drink (using Cannabis-Infused Milk, page 40) or your preferred dose (using a commercially made THC/CBD tincture of your choice)

EQUIPMENT:

Small saucepan

Whisk

Milk frother (optional)

Latte cup

INGREDIENTS:

1 cup (200 g) granulated sugar

1 cup (240 mL) water

¼ cup dried culinary lavender flowers

5 ounces (150 mL) milk of your choice (I prefer oat milk with this recipe)

2 ounces (60 mL) strong brewed coffee or espresso

¾ ounce (22 mL) lavender simple syrup

½ ounce (15 mL) Cannabis-Infused Milk (page 40)

Ground dried culinary lavender powder, for garnish

1 fresh lavender sprig, for garnish

1. To prepare the lavender syrup, add 1 cup (200 g) granulated sugar and 1 cup (240 mL) water to a small saucepan. Begin to heat over medium, constantly stirring until the sugar dissolves into the water.

2. Stir in the dried lavender, and bring to a soft boil for 1 minute. Remove from heat, and then steep for 30 minutes.

3. In a small saucepan, combine the milk of your choice with the brewed coffee and lavender simple syrup. Begin to warm over medium heat, stirring for 3 to 4 minutes or until hot (but not boiling).

4. When heated to your liking, remove from heat. Whisk in the Cannabis-Infused Milk.

5. Blend the ingredients together, creating a slight froth, and then remove from heat.

6. Pour the lavender latte into a latte cup, or use a whisk or milk frother to froth the latte even more.

7. Garnish with a dusting of ground dried lavender powder, for a boost of aromatics, and a lavender sprig.

> *Note:* **If you don't have the supplies to make the Cannabis-Infused Milk, simply skip this ingredient and add your favorite unflavored tincture (at your preferred dose) into the saucepan at step 4; whisk the ingredients together and then proceed with the recipe as noted. Just be sure to add ½ ounce (15 mL) of noninfused milk to keep the ratio the same. For the ground lavender powder, add 2 to 3 tablespoons dried culinary lavender to a coffee grinder. Grind until it forms a fine powder, and then add to a powdered sugar shaker before using.**

SWEET PEA CUCUMBER SOUR

Fresh from the garden, this Sweet Pea Cucumber Sour intertwines a bounty of botanicals that dazzle the senses. Don't forget to dry shake before adding ice for the best frothy outcome!

EQUIPMENT:

Saucepan

Fine-mesh strainer

Cheesecloth

Storage container of your choice

Shaker tin

Muddler

Hawthorne strainer

Chilled sour glass

Cocktail pick

INGREDIENTS:

1 cup (200 g) granulated sugar

1 cup (240 mL) water

¾ cup chopped sugar snap sweet peas

5 thick slices English cucumber, peeled and quartered

2 ounces (60 mL) freshly squeezed lime juice, pulp removed

1 ounce (30 mL) sweet pea simple syrup

1 ounce (30 mL) botanical gin

1 egg white

1 milliliter Cannabis-Infused Tincture (page 42)

Lime twist, for garnish

Sweet peas tendrils and floating seasonal flowers, for garnish

TARGET DOSE:

4 mg THC | < 1 mg CBD per milliliter per drink (using the Cannabis-Infused Tincture, page 42) or your preferred dose (using a commercially made THC/CBD tincture of your choice)

1. To prepare the sweet pea simple syrup, add 1 cup (200 g) granulated sugar and 1 cup (240 mL) water to a small saucepan. Begin to heat over medium, constantly stirring until the sugar dissolves into the water.

2. Stir in the chopped sugar snap sweet peas and bring to a boil. Promptly remove from heat, and let steep for 20 to 25 minutes or until you can taste the snap sweet pea flavor. When cooking, be careful not to overheat otherwise it will taste like bitter green beans!

3. Fine-strain the simple syrup through a fine-mesh strainer and cheesecloth into a cleaned storage container of your choice. Discard the solids.

4. In a shaker tin, muddle the cucumber and lime juice for 1 to 2 minutes to extract as much juice, color, and flavor as possible.

5. Fine-strain the liquid to remove the solids; then pour the liquid back into a clean shaker tin. Discard the solids.

6. Add the sweet pea simple syrup, gin, egg white, and Cannabis-Infused Tincture to the shaker tin. Dry shake (no ice) for 15 seconds; then add ice, and shake again for 20 seconds until very cold. Fine-strain into a chilled sour glass. Twist the lime peel over the glass to express the oils, then garnish. For extra flair, add fresh sweet pea tendrils and floating seasonal flowers, then enjoy immediately.

> *Note:* If you'd rather make this a mocktail, swap the gin for a nonalcoholic botanical gin and adjust the flavor as needed. See "Resources," on page 148, for a recommendation.

BUTTERFLY PEA BLACKBERRY ICED TEA

Glowing bright blue and purple, this magical iced tea enchants the senses. Although its deep color might appear to taste sweet, you may be surprised to discover that butterfly pea tea tastes slightly like green tea (and it's rich in antioxidants). The addition of citrus changes the pH of the tea, creating an array of purple, violet, and magenta colors and making this iced tea a tasty and beautiful concoction. The tea flavors are complemented by a touch of sweet and sour notes, which is why I love mixing it a little bit with honey, Cannabis-Infused Blackberry Simple Syrup, and freshly squeezed lemon juice.

TARGET DOSE:

10 to 11 mg THC | < 1 mg CBD per drink (using Cannabis-Infused Blackberry Simple Syrup, page 51) or your preferred dose (using a commercially made THC/CBD tincture of your choice)

EQUIPMENT:

Small saucepan

Rubber spatula

Fine-mesh strainer

16-ounce (480 mL) clean mason jar

Hawthorne strainer

Highball glass

Mixing glass

Bar spoon

INGREDIENTS:

8 ounces (240 mL) water

⅛ cup dried butterfly pea flowers

2½ teaspoons honey

6 ounces (180 mL) butterfly pea tea

¾ ounce (22 mL) Cannabis-Infused Blackberry Simple Syrup (page 51)

1¼ (37.5 mL) freshly squeezed lemon juice

Cubed ice

Lemon round, for garnish

Blackberries, for garnish

Floating butterfly pea flowers, for garnish

1. In a small saucepan, bring the water to a boil.

2. Remove from heat, and then add the butterfly pea flowers. Steep for 5 minutes or until the water has turned a dark blue color, gently stirring the leaves with a rubber spatula to extract the color.

3. When you've achieved a dark enough color, use a fine-mesh strainer to strain the liquids from the solids over a clean 16-ounce (480 mL) mason jar. Add the honey, stir to combine, and then let cool to room temperature.

4. In a mixing glass, add 6 ounces (180 mL) of the butterfly pea tea and Cannabis-Infused Blackberry Simple Syrup. Stir to combine, then pour into a highball glass filled with fresh ice. Slowly pour in the citrus and watch the colors change!

5. Stir the drink, and then garnish with a lemon round , blackberries, and floating butterfly pea flowers.

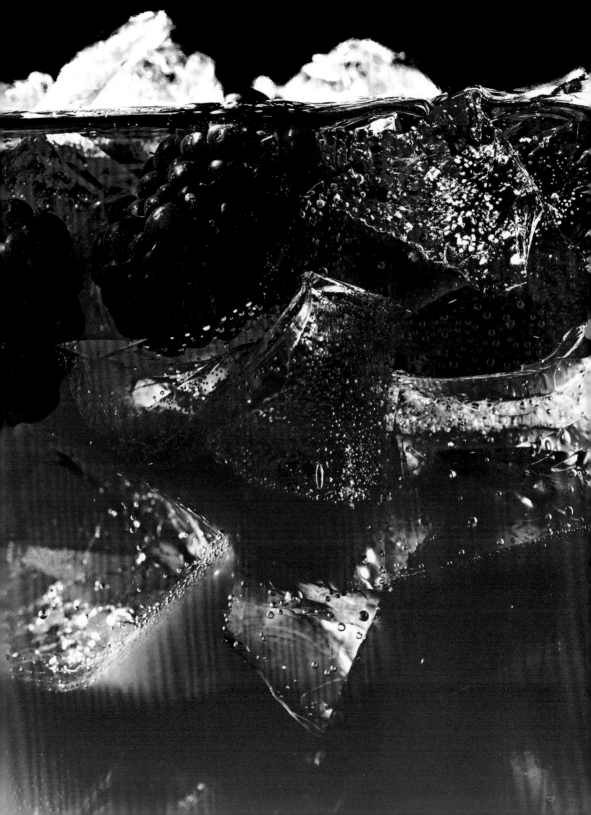

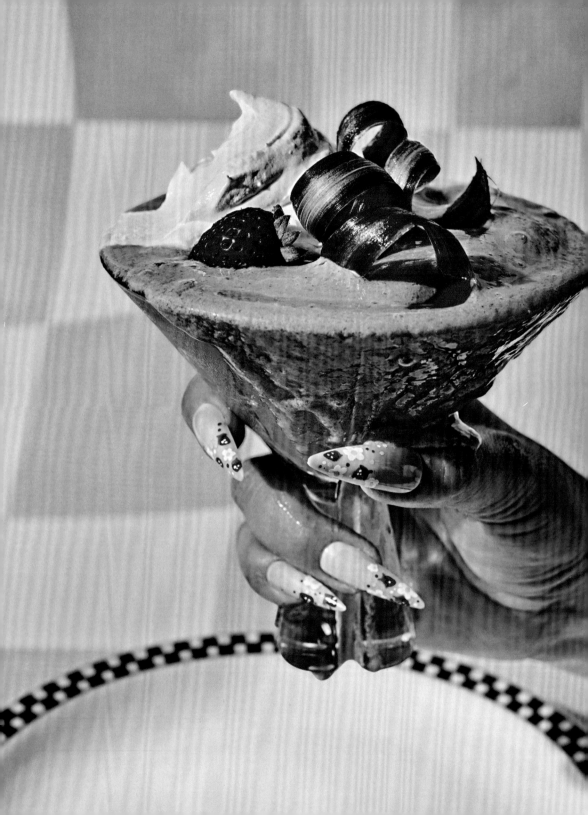

STRAWBERRY RHUBARB MILK SHAKE

If you're a fan of strawberry rhubarb pie, you're going to love this strawberry rhubarb milk shake! Made with all the right ingredients, including a dollop of strawberry rhubarb jam, this creamy shake is ideal when you're in the mood to celebrate spring flavors. For a boost of nutrition, I love adding a scoop of vanilla protein powder and a teaspoon of Cannabis-Infused Honey. Although I highly recommend trying this recipe as is, if you prefer to skip the extra sugar, simply swap the cannabis honey for your favorite unflavored tincture, and blend away (see note).

TARGET DOSE:

8 to 9 mg THC | < 3 mg CBD per drink (using Cannabis-Infused Honey, page 48) or your preferred dose (using a commercially made THC/CBD tincture of your choice)

EQUIPMENT:

Blender

Glass of your choice

INGREDIENTS:

1 cup frozen strawberries

½ cup frozen rhubarb

1 large frozen banana

6 ounces (180 mL) milk of your choice (I prefer oat milk with this shake)

1 scoop vanilla protein powder

2 teaspoons strawberry rhubarb jam (see "Resources," on page 148, for the kind I use)

1 teaspoon Cannabis-Infused Honey (page 48)

1 slice strawberry, for garnish

1 rhubarb ribbon, for garnish

Whipped cream, optional

1. Add all ingredients except the strawberry slice and the rhubarb ribbon to a blender.

2. Blend until smooth and creamy.

3. Serve in a glass of your choice, and top with the whipped cream (if using), the slice of strawberry, and the rhubarb ribbon.

> *Note:* **If you don't have time to make Cannabis-Infused Honey, you can still incorporate phytocannabinoids into this recipe by adding your favorite unflavored tincture (at your preferred dose) to the blender. Simply blend with the other ingredients called for in step 1, and enjoy.**

SPRING RECIPES

CARROT MULE

During the springtime, I love to make carrot drinks, especially when combined with ginger flavors. This healthy and refreshing combination quenches the thirst while providing a boost of nutrients and antioxidants. Fresh-pressed carrot juice and ginger can also help boost the immune system, making this nonalcoholic drink more than just a tasty concoction. If you're a fan of the Moscow mule, give this seasonal spin a try, and be sure to add fresh-pressed carrot juice for the healthiest benefits.

TARGET DOSE:

8 mg THC | 3 mg CBD per drink (using Cannabis-Infused Maple Syrup, page 54) or your preferred dose (using a commercially made THC/CBD tincture of your choice)

EQUIPMENT:

16-ounce (480 mL) copper mug

Bar spoon

Cocktail pick

INGREDIENTS:

4 ounces (120 mL) fresh-pressed carrot juice

½ ounce (15 mL) Cannabis-Infused Maple Syrup (page 54)

1½ ounces (45 mL) freshly squeezed lime juice

Ice to fill the mug (cracked iced is recommended, but cubed ice works, too)

Ginger beer (see "Resources," on page 148, for the brand I use)

Fresh carrot ribbon, for garnish

Fresh carrot greens, for garnish

1. Combine the carrot juice, Cannabis-Infused Maple Syrup, and lime juice in a copper mug; stir the ingredients well using a bar spoon.

2. Fill the mug with ice, and then top with ginger beer, slowly pouring until the mug is full.

3. Give the drink a stir, and then garnish with the carrot ribbon and carrot greens before serving.

Note: To make this drink a cocktail, simply add 1 ounce (30 mL) vodka to step 1 and follow the directions as noted.

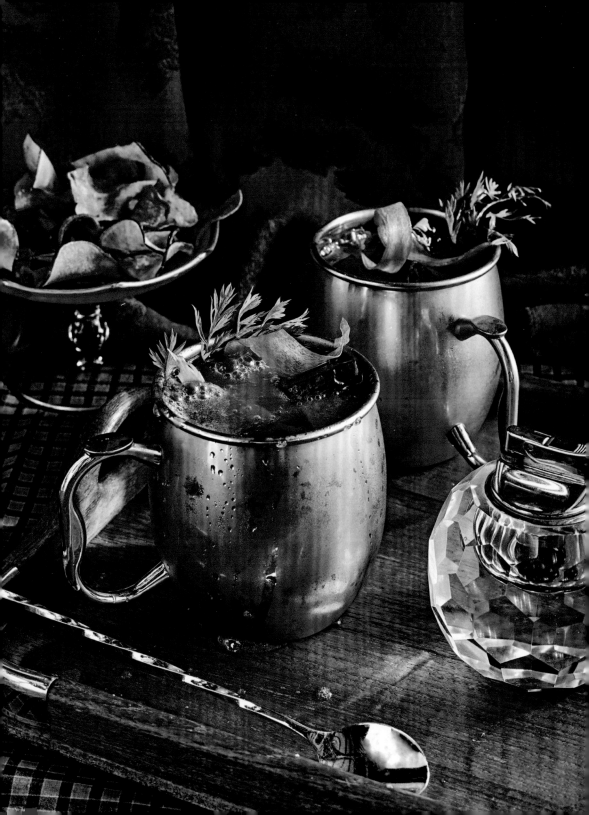

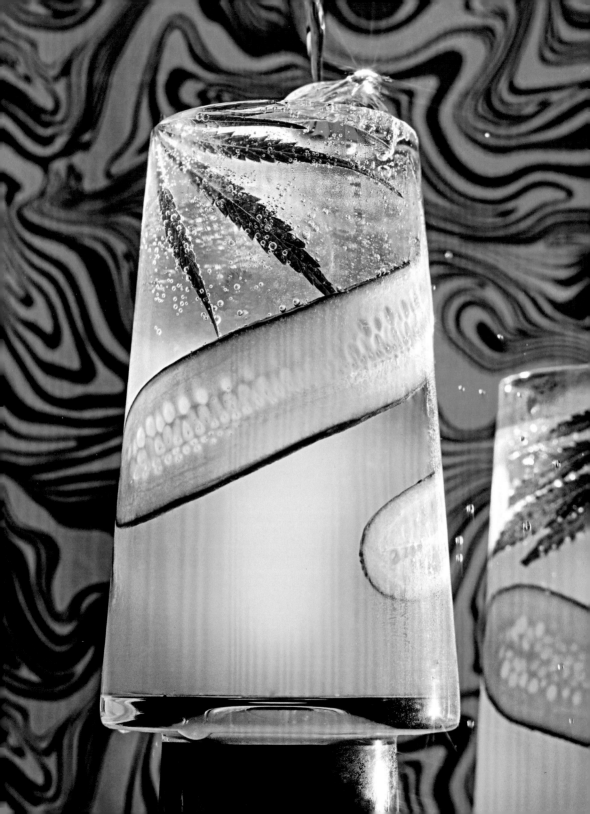

SEEDLING SPRITZ

Both floral and herbal, Lillet (pronounced lee-Lay) is one of my favorite French aromatized aperitifs. Made from Bordeaux grapes and fortified with a blend of liqueurs that have been flavored with different herbs, citrus, and botanicals, it's light and refreshing—a fantastic base for a spring spritz! With its herbaceous characteristics, it perfectly complements cannabis notes, making this your go-to spritz for the season.

TARGET DOSE:

8 mg THC | < 1 mg CBD per drink (using Cannabis-Infused Simple Syrup, page 49) or your preferred dose (using a commercially made THC/CBD tincture of your choice)

EQUIPMENT:

Shaker tin

Muddler

Fine-mesh strainer

Mixing glass

Bar spoon

Stemless wine glass

INGREDIENTS:

5 thick slices English cucumber, cut into quarters

1¼ ounce (37.5 mL) freshly squeezed lemon juice

½ ounce (15 mL) Cannabis-Infused Simple Syrup (page 49)

2 ounces (60 mL) Lillet Blanc (see note)

Cubed ice

2½ ounces (75 mL) chilled sparkling brut wine

2 ounces (60 mL) chilled club soda

1 to 2 cucumber ribbons and cannabis leaves (or other fresh garden herbs) wrapped around the inside of the glass

1. Combine the cucumber and lemon juice in a shaker tin.

2. Muddle the ingredients to extract as much cucumber juice and essence as possible. Fine-strain the liquid from the solids over a mixing glass. Add the cannabis-infused simple syrup and Lillet blanc, then stir to combine.

3. Pour the liquid into a stemless wine glass filled with fresh ice and garnish with a cucumber ribbon and cannabis leaves, wrapped inside of the glass. Discard the solids.

4. Add the sparkling brut wine and club soda, carefully stirring with a bar spoon to combine, then enjoy!

> *Note:* **If you'd rather skip the alcohol, you can swap the Lillet for a nonalcoholic botanical spirit made with botanical extracts and substitute the sparkling wine with additional club soda. Flip to the Resources on page 148 for my favorite kind.**

STRAWBERRY LEMONADE

Tart, sweet, and bright pink, this cannabis-infused Strawberry Lemonade is a go-to when you're craving something incredibly refreshing! Made with fresh strawberries and home-made lemonade that's been infused with cannabis simple syrup, this nonalcoholic recipe is ideal for those warm spring afternoons to quench your thirst. For the best strawberry flavor, you'll want to prepare strawberry purée, so be sure to have a blender or food processor handy. I also recommend making your own lemonade for this recipe, but if you're in a hurry, you can swap it for a store-bought variety.

TARGET DOSE:

8 mg THC | < 1 mg CBD per drink (using Cannabis-Infused Simple Syrup, page 49) or your preferred dose (using a commercially made THC/CBD tincture of your choice)

EQUIPMENT:

Single-serve blender

Fine-mesh strainer

Mixing bowl

Whisk

Highball glass (or glass of your choice)

INGREDIENTS:

5 large fresh strawberries (this purée should yield just under 4 ounces (120 mL), so save the rest for a second round)

4 ounces (120 mL) freshly squeezed lemon juice

2 ounces (60 mL) regular simple syrup

½ ounce (15 mL) Cannabis-Infused Simple Syrup (page 49)

4 ounces (120 mL) water

2 ounces (60 mL) strawberry purée

Cubed ice

1 small strawberry, for garnish

Lemon wheel, for garnish

1. Hull the strawberries, and add them to a single-serve blender or food processor. Purée for about 1 minute or until smooth.

2. Strain the strawberry purée through a fine-mesh strainer to remove the seeds; then set aside.

3. Add the lemon juice, simple syrup, Cannabis-Infused Simple Syrup, and water to a mixing bowl. Whisk together the lemonade. Taste, and adjust the flavor to your liking.

4. Combine the lemonade with the strawberry purée, and continue to whisk until combined well. Strain into a highball glass filled ¾ with fresh ice.

5. Garnish with the small strawberry and lemon wheel, and enjoy!

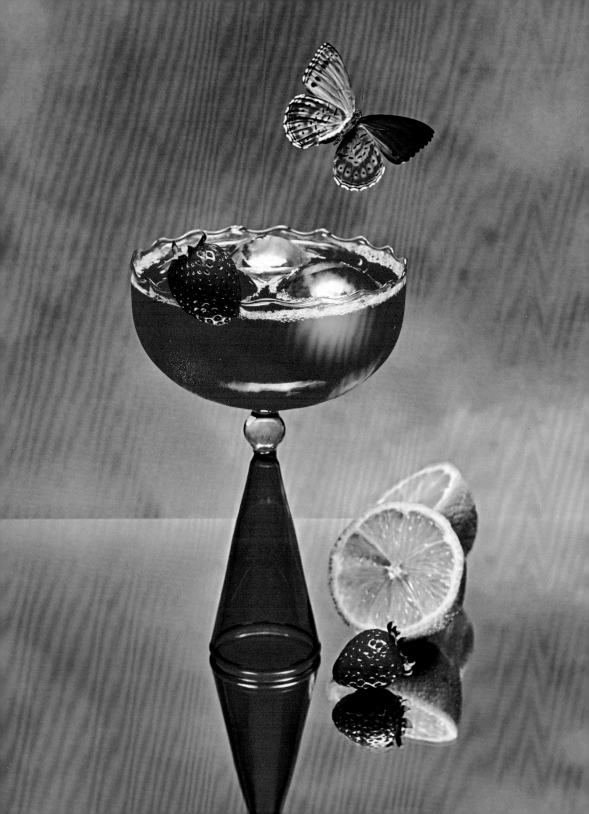

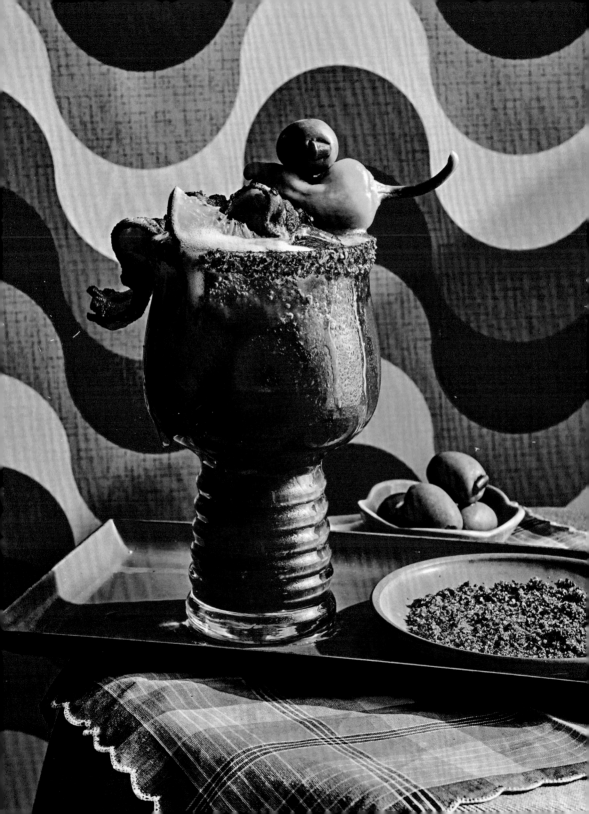

SPICY MEZCAL MICHELADA

Ideal for brunch and beyond, this drink is a perfect substitute for a Bloody Mary and offers some heightened ingredients to keep the good vibes flowing. This recipe differs from the standard michelada by including a splash of cannabis-infused Bacon Fat–Washed Mezcal and other flavorsome ingredients with a kick of heat! If you prefer a stronger dose, opt for the cannabis-infused salted chile rim.

TARGET DOSE:

6 to 7 mg THC | < 1 mg CBD per drink (using Bacon Fat–Washed Mezcal, page 46) or your preferred dose (using a commercially made nonalcoholic cannabis-infused beer, see note on following page)

EQUIPMENT:

Saucer

Boston shaker

Two 16-ounce (480 mL) clean mason jars

INGREDIENTS:

1 teaspoon Cannabis-Infused Salt (page 53—if you don't want to use infused salt, use regular salt)

1 teaspoon chile lime seasoning

Lime wedge

½ jalapeno, seeded and center removed

2 teaspoons hot sauce of your choice

1 ounce (30 mL) freshly squeezed lime juice

1 medium pepperoncini, stemmed

¼ teaspoon prepared horseradish

Dash cumin

Dash salt

Dash black pepper

Dash celery salt

5 ounces (150 mL) tomato juice (see "Resources," on page 148, for the kind I use)

1½ ounces (45 mL) spicy sauce

½ ounce (15 mL) freshly squeezed lime juice

½ ounce (15 mL) cannabis-infused Bacon Fat–Washed Mezcal (page 46)

1 teaspoon pimiento-stuffed manzanilla olive juice

1 or 2 dashes Worcestershire sauce

Cubed ice

Light Mexican beer (see "Resources," on page 148, for the kind I use)

Peppered bacon, for garnish

Stuffed manzanilla olives, for garnish

Lime wedge, for garnish

CONTINUED ON PAGE 76

I. Combine the Cannabis-Infused Salt (if using) and chile lime seasoning in a small saucer. Rim the top of the glass with a lime wedge, and then dip the top of the glass into the chile lime seasoning to create a salted rim. Set the glass aside.

2. Next, create the spicy sauce. Add the jalapeño, hot sauce, lime juice, pepperoncini, horserad-ish, cumin, salt, pepper, and celery salt to a single-serve blender. Blend on high until smooth. Set aside.

3. In a Boston shaker, add the tomato juice, 1½ ounces (45 mL) spicy sauce, freshly squeezed lime juice, Bacon Fat–Washed Mezcal, olive juice, and Worcestershire sauce in one part of the shaker.

4. To best mix the ingredients together, you'll want to "roll" the liquid instead of shaking or stirring. To do so, fill a clean 16-ounce (480 mL) mason jar three-quarters of the way full of ice to accurately measure, and then pour the ice into the other part of the Boston shaker. Pour the liquid ingredients over the ice, and then roll the liquid back and forth between both shakers about four times to mix the ingredients.

5. After mixing well, pour the liquid and ice into the salted 16-ounce mason jar, and top with the beer. Stir to combine, and garnish with a piece of peppered bacon, stuffed manzanilla olives, and a lime wedge.

6. Serve immediately, and enjoy this tasty and savory beverage!

Note: **If you'd rather skip the alcohol in this recipe, you can still prepare the michelada by incorporating your choice of nonalcoholic cannabis-infused beer. This will also guarantee a precise dose. See "Resources," on page 148, for my favorite kind.**

RHUBARB SPARKLER

When you're in the mood for an effervescent, easy-drinking pink drink, look no further than this Rhubarb Sparkler! If you can't find fresh rhubarb to make the syrup, frozen rhubarb works fine—it just might not be as pink (or tart).

TARGET DOSE:

7 to 8 mg THC | 1 mg CBD per drink (using Cannabis-Infused Sugar, page 55, and Cannabis-Infused Tincture, page 42) or your preferred dose (using a commercially made THC/CBD tincture of your choice)

INGREDIENTS:

2 cups rhubarb, chopped into pieces

2 cups (480 mL) water

1 cup (200 g) sugar

1 teaspoon Cannabis-Infused Sugar (page 55)

Lemon wedge

1½ ounces (45 mL) rhubarb syrup

⅓ cup fresh raspberries

1½ ounces (45 mL) freshly squeezed lemon juice

1 milliliter Cannabis-Infused Tincture (page 42)

Cubed ice

Club soda

1 rhubarb ribbon, for garnish

EQUIPMENT:

Saucepan

Fine-mesh strainer

Mixing spoon

Funnel

Airtight swing bottle or storage container of your choice

Saucer

Rocks glass

Shaker tin

Muddler

Fine-mesh strainer

Bar spoon

Cocktail pick

1. To prepare the rhubarb syrup, heat the chopped rhubarb and water in a medium saucepan. Reduce to medium heat, and simmer for 25 to 30 minutes or until the water has absorbed most of the pink pigment. Remove from heat.

2. Use a fine-mesh strainer to separate the rhubarb solids from the liquid, and discard the cooked rhubarb.

3. Add the rhubarb-infused water to a clean saucepan, and begin to heat again. Add the granulated sugar, and begin to stir until all the sugar has dissolved. Remove from heat, and let cool to room temperature. Once cooled, funnel the liquid into an airtight swing bottle, and set aside.

4. In a small saucer, add the Cannabis-Infused Sugar. Rim the top of a rocks glass with a lemon wedge, and then dip the edge of the glass into the sugar to create an infused-sugar rim. Set aside.

5. In a shaker tin, muddle the rhubarb syrup and raspberries until they release their juices.

6. Add the lemon juice, Cannabis-Infused Tincture, and ice. Cover and shake for 15 seconds or until very cold; then fine-strain into a rocks glass filled with fresh ice.

7. Top with club soda, and give the drink a few good stirs using a bar spoon.

8. Garnish with a rhubarb ribbon on a cocktail pick, and enjoy!

FORBIDDEN FRUIT FIZZ

If you're a fan of a Ramos Gin Fizz, you're going to love this Forbidden Fruit Fizz! Inspired by the mesmerizing aromas and flavors of the cannabis strain Forbidden Fruit, which is a cross of Cherry Pie and Tangie, this fizzy and fruity nonalcoholic drink will excite your senses. Combining fresh tangerine juice, cherry juice, lime juice, fresh raspberries, homemade Cannabis-Infused Grenadine Syrup, egg whites, and club soda, this sumptuous recipe is great for when you're in the mood for something exotic.

TARGET DOSE:

3 to 4 mg THC | < 1 mg CBD per drink (using Cannabis-Infused Grenadine Syrup, page 56) or your preferred dose (using a commercially made THC/CBD tincture of your choice)

EQUIPMENT:

Shaker tin

Muddler

Fine-mesh strainer

Hawthorne strainer

Chilled rocks glass

Cocktail pick

INGREDIENTS:

⅓ cup fresh raspberries

2 ounces (60 mL) fresh tangerine juice (substitute orange juice if you can't find tangerine)

1¼ ounces (37.5 mL) tart cherry juice (see "Resources," on page 148, for the kind I use)

1 ounce (30 mL) fresh lime juice

¾ ounce (22 mL) Cannabis-Infused Grenadine Syrup (page 53)

1 egg white

Cubed iced

Splash of club soda

1 cannabis leaf, for garnish

1 orange twist, for garnish

Raspberries, for garnish

I. In a shaker tin, add the raspberries, tangerine juice, cherry juice, and lime juice. Muddle the ingredients until the raspberry juices release.

2. Use a fine-mesh strainer to separate the liquid, and discard the solids.

3. Pour the liquid back into a cleaned shaker tin, and then add the Cannabis-Infused Grenadine Syrup and egg white. Cover the shaker tin, and dry shake vigorously (no ice) for about 15 seconds. Add ice, and shake again until very cold.

4. Using a Hawthorne strainer, strain the liquid through a fine-mesh strainer into a chilled rocks glass filled with fresh cubed ice. Shake the shaker tin and strainer to get as much foam as possible.

5. Top with a splash of club soda, gently stir, and then garnish with a cannabis leaf, an orange twist, and raspberries speared on a cocktail pick.

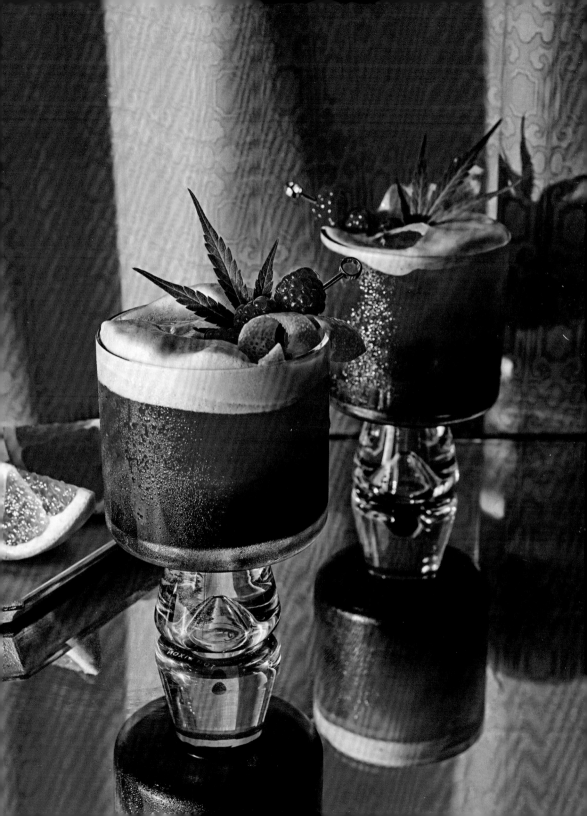

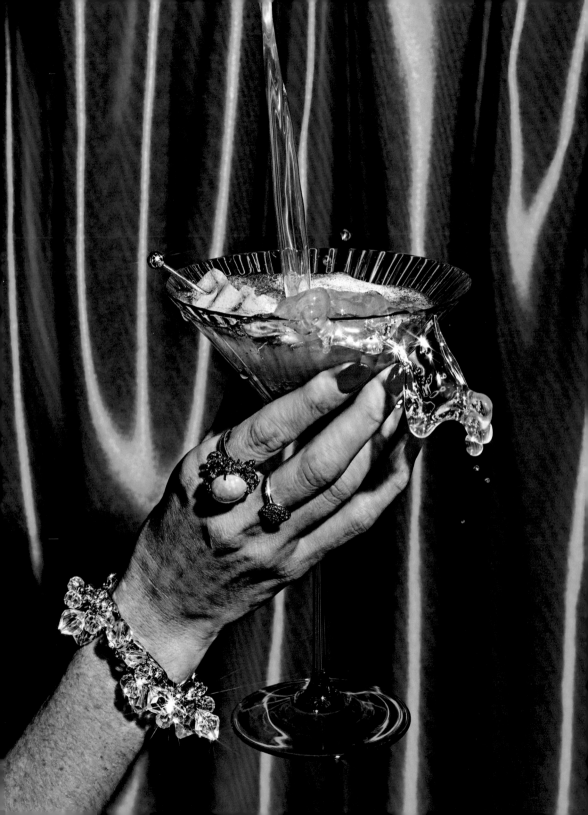

BUMBLE BEE'S KNEES

During springtime, bees work their magic, spreading pollen to flowering plants and crops. To honor their hard work, this infused Bumble Bee's Knees is the ultimate celebration! If you're a fan of the classic Bee's Knees cocktail (which originated during the 1920s, thanks to Margaret Brown—the "Unsinkable Molly Brown," who survived the *Titanic* disaster), this infused version combines all the traditional ingredients, except that you'll be adding Cannabis-Infused Honey Simple Syrup (page 49) to elevate the cocktail.

TARGET DOSE:

8 mg THC | < 1 mg CBD per drink (using Cannabis-Infused Honey Simple Syrup, page 49) or your preferred dose (using a commercially made cannabis-infused honey—see the accompanying note)

EQUIPMENT:

Shaker tin

Coupe glass

INGREDIENTS:

2 ounces (60 mL) gin (see the accompanying note for the style of gin to use)

¾ ounce (22 mL) freshly squeezed lemon juice

¾ ounce (22 mL) Cannabis-Infused Honey Simple Syrup, page 49

Lemon twist, for garnish

1. In a cocktail shaker tin, add the gin, lemon juice, and Cannabis-Infused Honey Simple Syrup. Fill the shaker tin halfway with ice, cover the shaker, and then shake vigorously for 25 to 30 seconds or until very cold. A proper shake will allow for the appropriate dilution.

2. Strain the liquid into a chilled coupe glass, and then add the lemon twist over the glass to express the citrus oils before garnishing.

3. Serve immediately, and enjoy!

> *Note:* **For the best flavor, you'll want to use a gin that's been slightly sweetened with honey. Flip to "Resources," on page 148, for the kind I use—it's the perfect match for this recipe! If you'd rather skip the alcohol, you can use a nonalcoholic gin substitute. You can also get creative and incorporate a nonalcoholic cannabis-infused spirit or simply use a noninfused honey simple syrup.**

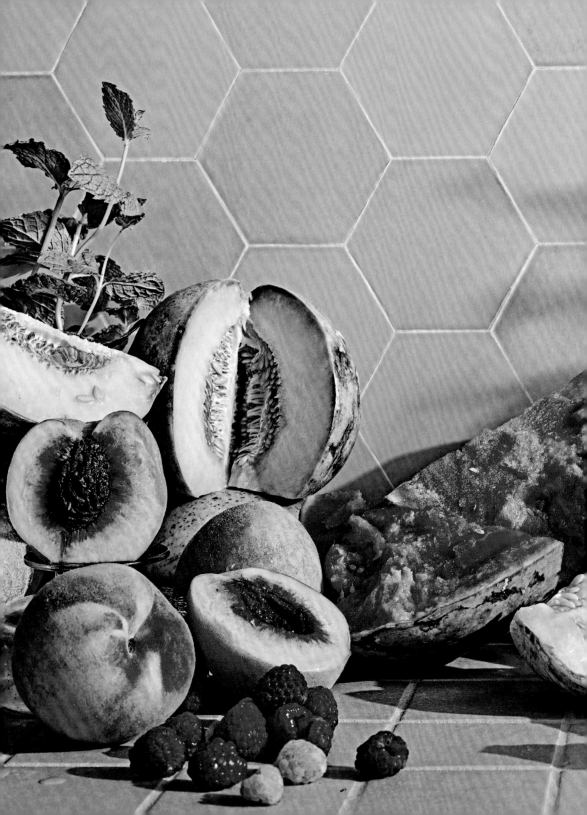

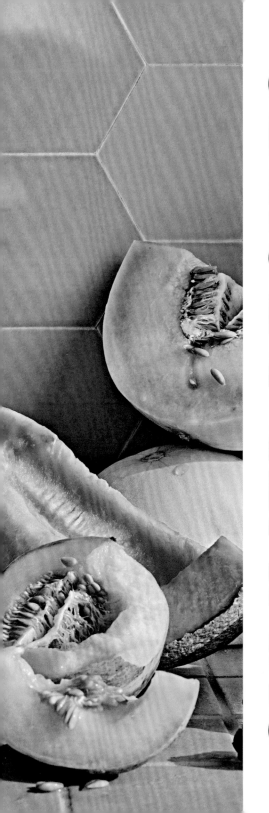

SUMMER RECIPES

CHAPTER 4

Summer is the ultimate time of year to celebrate the freshest fruit flavors. As temperatures begin to rise, refreshing drinks are top of mind, which means our palates crave everything and anything chilled. In this chapter, you discover the refreshing flavors that are best enjoyed during those long summer days. Perfect for poolside sipping or backyard barbeques with friends, this collection of cool, mouthwatering drinks is meant to keep you high and hydrated, so I hope you're feeling thirsty!

SUN-KISSED SUMMER JUICE

During the warmer months, there's nothing better than fruits and veggies fresh from the garden—particularly berries and summer beets! This delicious and nutritious juice will brighten up your day and provide plenty of antioxidants and vitamins to keep the body in balance. In addition to beets and berries, I love adding fresh citrus juice and a hint of ginger for an instant mood boost, along with chilled coconut water to provide extra hydration. Cheers to a healthy summer!

TARGET DOSE:

Nonintoxicating THCA and CBDA

EQUIPMENT:

Juicer

Mixing glass

Whisk

Glass of your choice

INGREDIENTS:

1 large red beet, peeled and quartered

1 cup fresh strawberries, stemmed and halved

1 cup fresh raspberries

1 cup fresh blackberries

1 chilled lemon, peeled and quartered

One 1-inch piece fresh ginger, peeled and sliced in half (add more if you love fresh ginger)

1 milliliter cannabis-infused fresh flower tincture (page 43)

1½ teaspoons blue agave syrup (adjust based on your preferred level of sweetness)

1 ounce (30 mL) chilled coconut water (see "Resources," on page 148, for the kind I use)

1. Feed the beets, strawberries, raspberries, blackberries, lemon, and ginger into a juicer, alternating the ingredients as you continue to juice.

2. Once everything is juiced, stir to combine; then transfer into a mixing glass. Add the cannabis-infused fresh flower tincture and coconut water, and whisk to combine.

3. Serve immediately, and enjoy with or without ice—your choice!

> *Note:* **Red beets can stain, so don't wear your favorite outfit when preparing this recipe.**

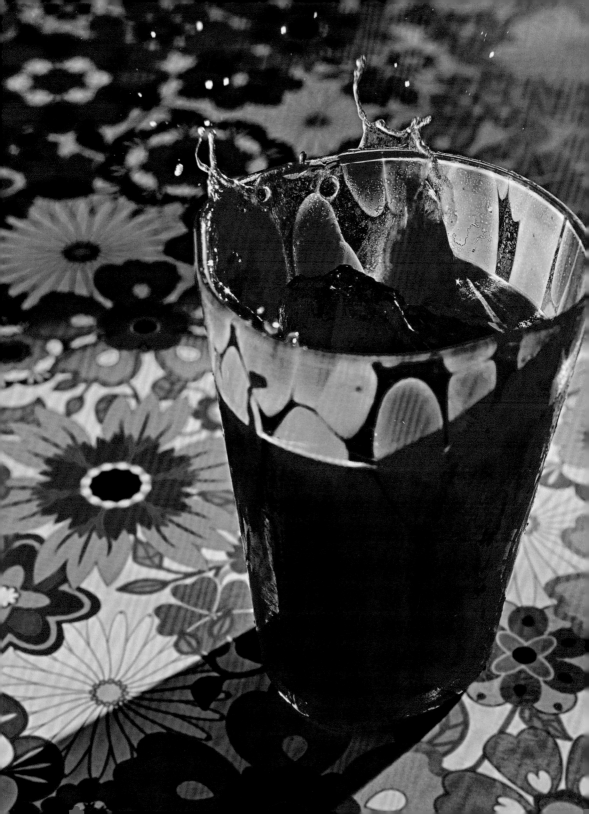

ICED CANNA-COFFEE

When it's hot outside and you need a boost of energy, look no further than this mouthwatering iced canna-coffee recipe. Different than other iced coffee drinks, this delectable, caffeinated beverage combines your favorite coffee and cream (or milk) with Cannabis-Infused Coffee Syrup and a hint of coconut extract. This deliciously dank combination is incredibly easy to prepare, as long as you have the infused coffee syrup prepared ahead of time (see page 52). If you'd like to increase the dosage and have some Cannabis-Infused Milk on hand, feel free to substitute it for a portion of the half-and-half that's called for.

TARGET DOSE:

6 to 7 mg THC | < 1 mg CBD per drink (using Cannabis-Infused Coffee Syrup, page 52) or your preferred dose (using a commercially made THC/CBD tincture of your choice)

EQUIPMENT:

Boston shaker

Highball glass

Reusable straw

INGREDIENTS:

8 ounces (240 mL) of your favorite strong coffee (at room temperature)

1 ounce (30 mL) half-and-half, or milk of your choice

¾ ounce (22 mL) Cannabis-Infused Coffee Syrup (page 52—adjust depending on your dosage and sweet preference)

½ teaspoon coconut extract

Cubed ice

1. In a Boston shaker, add the coffee, half-and-half, Cannabis-Infused Coffee Syrup, and coconut extract in one part of the shaker.

2. To best mix the ingredients together, you'll want to "roll" the liquid instead of stirring (or shaking), which will also add a slight froth. To do so, fill a clean highball glass with cubed ice; then pour the ice into the other part of the Boston shaker. Pour the liquid ingredients over the ice, and roll the liquid back and forth between both shakers about three times to mix the ingredients.

3. After mixing well, pour the liquid and ice into the highball glass, add a reusable straw, and enjoy!

BASIL BERRY ICED TEA

Blackberry, strawberry, and basil. What an epic combination of flavors, especially in summer! During those long, hot days, this easy-to-make iced tea will keep your palate chilled and refreshed while providing a healthy dose of phytocannabinoids. You want the berry and basil flavors to shine in this recipe, so it's recommended to use a more neutral tea (such as green tea) to complement the other ingredients in this recipe and provide some uplifting caffeine.

TARGET DOSE:

10 to 11 mg THC | < 1 mg CBD per drink (using Cannabis-Infused Blackberry Simple Syrup, page 51) or your preferred dose (using a commercially made THC/CBD tincture of your choice)

EQUIPMENT:

Small saucepan

16-ounce (480 mL) clean mason jar

Bar spoon

Muddler

> *Note:* **Flip to "Resources," on page 148, for the green tea I use for this recipe (1 tea bag per cup).**

INGREDIENTS:

8 ounces (240 mL) water

1 green tea bag

1 teaspoon honey

5 to 6 fresh basil leaves

¼ cup fresh blackberries

¼ cup strawberries, stemmed and quartered

1 ounce (30 mL) lemon juice

Cubed Ice

5 ounces (150 mL) green tea, at room temperature (see the accompanying note)

¾ ounce (22 mL) Cannabis-Infused Blackberry Simple Syrup (page 51)

1 teaspoon blue agave syrup (add more if you prefer a sweeter tea)

Basil sprig, for garnish

1 strawberry slice, for garnish

Blackberries, for garnish

Seasonal edible flowers, for garnish

1. In a small saucepan, heat the water until warm. Remove from heat, and add the green tea bag. Steep for 3 minutes, remove the tea bag, and discard; then add the honey. Stir to combine, and then let cool to room temperature.

2. Smack the basil leaves in your hands, to release the aromas; then place them in the bottom of a mason jar along with the blackberries, strawberries, and lemon juice.

3. Muddle the ingredients to release the berry juices and basil oils. For optimal results, be careful not to tear the leaves.

4. Fill the glass with ice, and then top with the green tea, Cannabis-Infused Blackberry Simple Syrup, and blue agave syrup. Using a bar spoon, stir to mix all ingredients.

5. Garnish with a basil sprig, floating blackberries, and seasonal edible flowers.

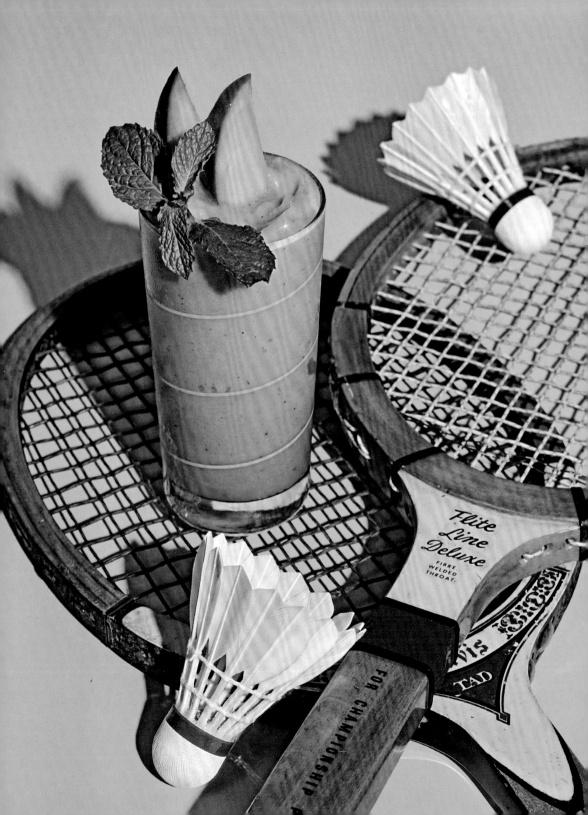

YIELD: 1 SERVING

MANGO TANGO SMOOTHIE

Inspired by the cannabis strain Mango Tango, this healthy smoothie combines the refreshing flavors of mango, peach, tangerine, and minty green goodness. Get ready to eat this with a spoon—it's thick and filling! Mangoes are rich in nutrients and contain high levels of vitamins, minerals, and antioxidants. Peaches and bananas are also good sources of fiber, making this smoothie a fantastic option for breakfast. Add a teaspoon of Cannabis-Infused Honey (or more, depending on your sweetness/dosage preferences), to easily enhance this recipe.

TARGET DOSE:

9 mg THC | 3 mg CBD per drink (using Cannabis-Infused Honey, page 48) or your preferred dose (using a commercially made THC/CBD tincture of your choice —see the accompanying note)

EQUIPMENT:

Blender

Glass of your choice

INGREDIENTS:

¾ cup frozen mango

½ cup frozen peaches

⅓ cup frozen pineapple

1 small frozen banana

6 ounces (180 mL) freshly squeezed tangerine juice (or substitute orange juice)

1 teaspoon Cannabis-Infused Honey (page 48)

1 teaspoon freshly squeezed lime juice

3 fresh mint leaves

Mint sprig, for garnish

Slice of fresh mango, for garnish

1. Add all the ingredients to a blender.

2. Blend until smooth and creamy.

3. Serve in a glass of your choice, and garnish with a mint sprig and a slice of fresh mango.

Note: If you haven't made the Cannabis-Infused Honey, you can still incorporate phytocannabinoids into this recipe by adding your favorite unflavored tincture (at your preferred dose) to the blender. Simply blend with the other ingredients, and enjoy.

FROZEN CHERRY LIMEADE

To beat the summer heat, this frozen cherry limeade is ice cold and will thoroughly keep you chilled. Be sure to use freshly squeezed lime juice for this recipe (never store bought); fresh lime juice presents the brightest citrus notes, which makes this drink oh-so-refreshing!

TARGET DOSE:

8 mg THC | < 1 mg CBD per drink (using Cannabis-Infused Simple Syrup, page 49) or your preferred dose (using a commercially made THC/CBD tincture of your choice—see the accompanying note)

EQUIPMENT:

Mixing glass

Bar spoon

Blender

Glass of your choice

INGREDIENTS:

4¾ ounces (142 mL) freshly squeezed lime juice

¾ ounce (22 mL) regular simple syrup

½ ounce (15 mL) Cannabis-Infused Simple Syrup (page 49)

1 cup frozen cherries (I used a triple cherry blend)

1 cup ice

Lime wheel, for garnish

Fresh cherries, for garnish

I. To make the limeade, add the lime juice, simple syrup, and Cannabis-Infused Simple Syrup to a mixing glass. Stir to combine (feel free to adjust the flavor, if it's too tart for your preference).

2. Combine the limeade, frozen cherries, and ice in the bottom of a blender.

3. Blend until smooth, and then pour into a glass of your choice.

4. Garnish with a lime wheel and fresh cherries on top.

> *Tip!* If you prefer a thicker frozen drink, prepare the limeade ahead of time, and then freeze the juice into ice cubes. Once frozen, add the frozen limeade ice cubes, frozen cherries, and ice to the blender in step 1, and follow the directions as noted.

> *Note:* If you don't have time to prepare the Cannabis-Infused Simple Syrup, you can still incorporate phytocannabinoids into this recipe by adding your favorite unflavored tincture (at your preferred dose) to the blender. Simply blend with the other ingredients, and enjoy.

PEACH BELLINI POPSICLES

This tasty summer treat can be enjoyed as a straight-up popsicle, or if you're feeling a little adventurous, you can combine it with prosecco rosé in a glass to make a popsicle cocktail. When you're craving a taste of summer, give these popsicles a try, and be sure to enjoy them with friends!

TARGET DOSE:

10 mg THC | 1 mg CBD per popsicle (using Cannabis-Infused Honey Simple Syrup, page 49) or your preferred dose (using a commercially made THC/CBD tincture of your choice)

EQUIPMENT:

Blender

Popsicle mold

Popsicle sticks

Mug

Wine glass

INGREDIENTS:

2 cups frozen peaches

1 ounce (30 mL) freshly squeezed lemon juice

3½ ounces (105 mL) Cannabis-Infused Honey Simple Syrup (page 49)

1 ounce (30 mL) filtered water

2½ ounces (75 mL) prosecco rosé—split between all (see "Resources," on page 148, for the kind I use)

1. Prepare the popsicles by adding the peaches, lemon juice, and Cannabis-Infused Honey Simple Syrup, and water to a blender. Blend on high, and then pour the liquified ingredients into the popsicle molds. This is the infused portion of the popsicle, so spreading evenly is key to ensure that the dosage is as accurate as possible.

2. Next, pour a splash of the prosecco rosé on top of the peach mix, and give it a stir using a popsicle stick. Once mixed, insert the popsicle sticks, and freeze overnight.

3. The next day, remove the pops from the molds. If you're having trouble removing the pop, fill a mug with room temperature water, and then dip each mold into the water for a few seconds to help slide out the popsicles. Immediately wash the molds, and create another batch, if needed.

4. You can enjoy this delicious popsicle as is or, for a fun drink, add the popsicles to a wine glass and top with prosecco rosé to make a popsicle rosé bellini cocktail!

> *Tip!* This popsicle tastes like a traditional bellini, but if you prefer a sweeter taste, add a few teaspoons of noninfused honey to the blender until you find your perfect flavor.

> *Note:* If you'd rather skip the alcohol, simply swap the prosecco for your favorite sparkling cannabis-infused drink that will blend well with peachy flavors. Just be sure to use noninfused honey simple syrup so that you're not double dosing. If you're not planning to enjoy these popsicles right away, the best way to store them is to wrap them in cellophane bags and then store them in a zip-top freezer bag, to prevent freezer burn.

CANTALOUPE AGUA FRESCA

Nothing screams *hydration* quite like a Cantaloupe Agua Fresca! This beyond-refreshing drink is designed to quench your thirst and is much lighter than typical juice because it contains coconut water and a touch of lime juice to brighten the flavor. I love adding fresh mint leaves for an even more refreshing drinking experience.

TARGET DOSE:

8 mg THC | < 1 mg CBD per drink (using Cannabis-Infused Simple Syrup, page 49) or your preferred dose (using a commercially made THC/CBD tincture of your choice)

EQUIPMENT:

Blender

Fine-mesh strainer

8-ounce (240 mL) clean mason jar

Highball glass

Muddler

Bar spoon

Cocktail pick

INGREDIENTS:

½ cantaloupe melon (save the other half of the melon for the garnish—and to snack on!)

4 ounces (120 mL) chilled coconut water

5 to 6 fresh mint leaves

1½ ounces (45 mL) freshly squeezed lime juice

½ ounce (15 mL) Cannabis-Infused Simple Syrup (page 49)

Cubed ice

6 ounces (180 mL) cantaloupe juice

Mint sprig, for garnish

Slice of cantaloupe, for garnish

1. To make the cantaloupe juice, place the cantaloupe flesh and coconut water into a blender or food processor. Purée for 1 minute or until the cantaloupe chunks liquify. Using a fine-mesh strainer, separate the pulp from the juice over an 8-ounce (240 mL) mason jar. Discard the pulp, and set the jar aside.

2. Smack the mint leaves in your hand to release the aromas, and then add them to the bottom of a highball glass along with the lime juice and Cannabis-Infused Simple Syrup. Muddle the ingredients until the mint oils release, being careful not to tear the leaves.

3. Fill the highball glass with cubed ice, and then top the drink wth 6 ounces of the cantaloupe juice. Stir with a bar spoon to combine; garnish with a mint sprig and a slice of cantaloupe, for garnish

4. Serve immediately, and enjoy!

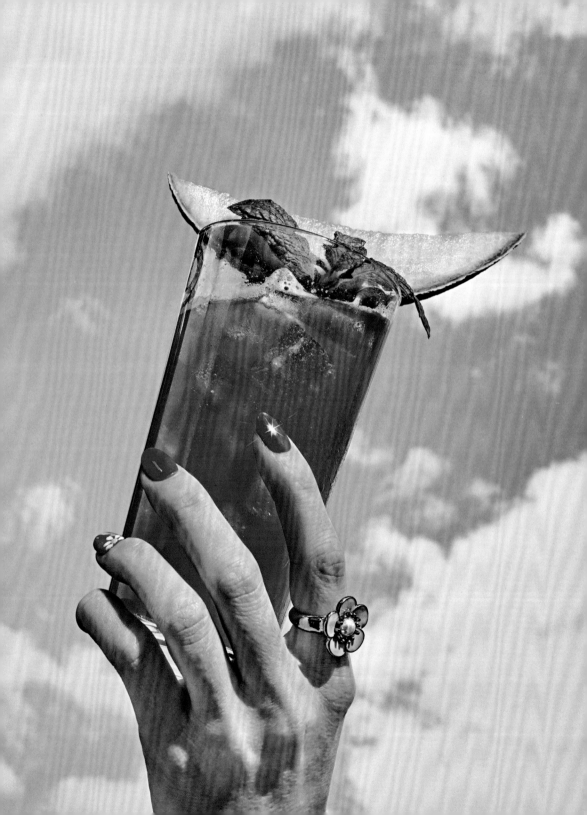

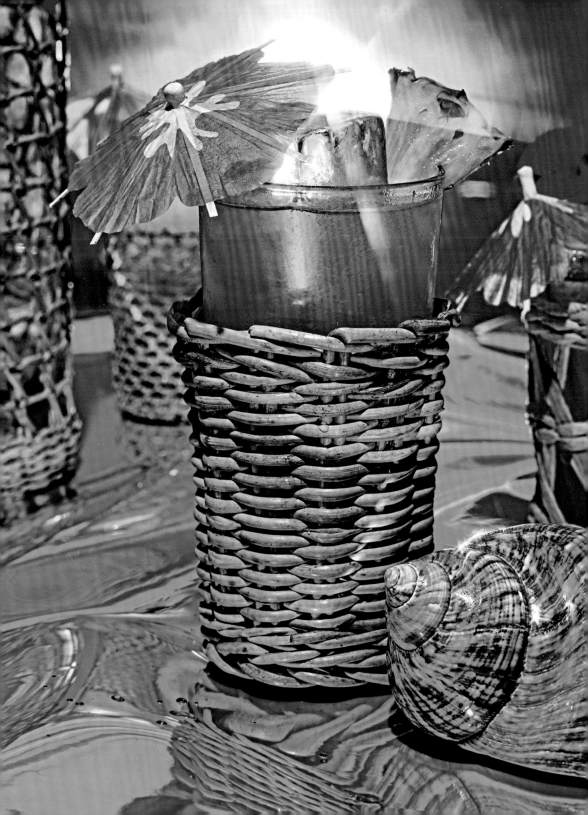

TROPICAL CANNA-COOLER

Calling all tropical fruit lovers! Treat your palate to a mini island vacation with this out-of-this-world refreshing drink. Both hydrating and delicious, this easy-to-make recipe is ideal for those hot summer days when you need something to cool you down. Combining pineapple juice with passion fruit juice, guava juice, lime juice, a cannabis-infused tincture, and a splash of coconut water, this drink belongs poolside—and it even comes with a mini drink umbrella!

TARGET DOSE:

4 to 8 mg THC | < 1 to 1 mg CBD per milliliter per drink (using the Cannabis-Infused Tincture, page 42) or your preferred dose (using a commercially made THC/CBD tincture of your choice)

EQUIPMENT:

Shaker tin

Highball glass

Hawthorne strainer

Mini drink umbrella

INGREDIENTS:

2½ ounces (75 mL) pineapple juice

2 ounces (60 mL) guava juice

1½ ounces (45 mL) passion fruit juice (see note)

1¼ ounces (37.5 mL) freshly squeezed lime juice

1 to 2 milliliters Cannabis-Infused Tincture (page 42)

Cubed ice

2 ounces (60 mL) coconut water

Pineapple leaf, for garnish

Pineapple slice, for garnish

Seasonal edible flowers, for garnish

1. In a shaker tin, combine the pineapple juice, guava juice, passion fruit juice, lime juice, and Cannabis-Infused Tincture.

2. Add ice, cover the shaker, and then shake for 10 seconds or until cold.

3. Strain into a highball glass filled to the top with fresh cubed ice, and then top with coconut water.

4. Stir to combine. Garnish with a pineapple leaf, a slice of pineapple, seasonal edible flowers, and a mini drink umbrella.

> *Note:* **The best passion fruit juice to use is cold-pressed instead of "naturally flavored" passion fruit juice from concentrate, which is packed with sugar. Flip to "Resources," on page 148, for the kind I love to mix with!**

HONEYDEW MELON MARGARITA

Light, refreshing, and glowing with a green hue, this Honeydew Melon Margarita is oh-so-tasty! The secret to this recipe is sourcing a perfectly ripe honeydew melon, to capture all of its essence. You'll also want to save a portion of the honeydew to garnish the drink, so be sure to set some aside (even though, if you're a honeydew lover like me, you may be tempted to eat it!). For an enhancement, rim the glass with Cannabis-Infused Salt and lime zest, to add a nice salty-sour combination to this recipe.

TARGET DOSE:

8 mg THC | < 1 mg CBD per drink (using Cannabis-Infused Simple Syrup, page 49, and Cannabis-Infused Salt, page 53) or your preferred dose (using a commercially made THC/CBD tincture of your choice)

EQUIPMENT:

Blender or food processor

Fine-mesh strainer

16-ounce (480 mL) sterilized mason jar

Saucer

Rocks glass

Shaker tin

Hawthorne strainer

Melon baller

Cocktail pick

INGREDIENTS:

½ medium honeydew melon (should yield about 1⅓ cups juice, so save the extra juice for more rounds)

Lime wedge

1 teaspoon Cannabis-Infused Salt (page 53)

Grated lime zest

3 ounces (90 mL) honeydew melon juice

1¾ ounces (52 mL) freshly squeezed lime juice

½ ounce (15 mL) Cannabis-Infused Simple Syrup (page 49)

1 ounce (30 mL) tequila blanco

1 large ice cube

Lime twist, for garnish

Honeydew melon balls on a cocktail pick, for garnish

Fresh cannabis leaves, for garnish

I. Begin by making the honeydew melon juice. Place the honeydew flesh into a blender or food processor. Purée for 1 minute or until the honeydew chunks turn into juice. Using a fine-mesh strainer, separate the pulp from the juice over a 16-ounce (480 mL) mason jar. Discard the pulp, and set the jar aside.

2. Next, create the salted rim. Add the Cannabis-Infused Salt to a small saucer. Rim a rocks glass with a lime wedge, and then dip the top of the glass into the salt. Set aside.

3. Add the honeydew melon juice, lime juice, Cannabis-Infused Simple Syrup, and tequila blanco to a shaker tin. Add ice, cover, and then shake for 20 seconds or until very cold.

4. Fill the salted glass with one large ice cube. Strain the drink into the glass.

5. Garnish with a lime twist, honeydew melon balls on a cocktail pick, and fresh cannabis leaves; then enjoy!

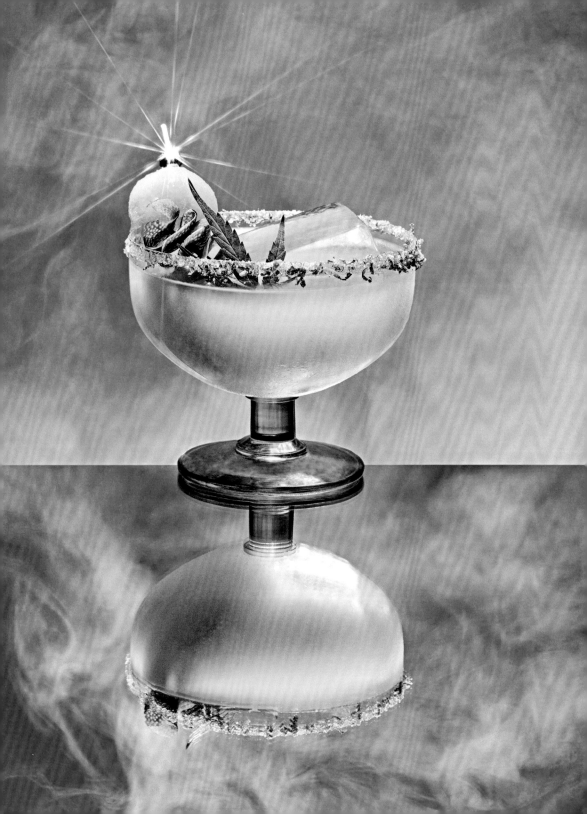

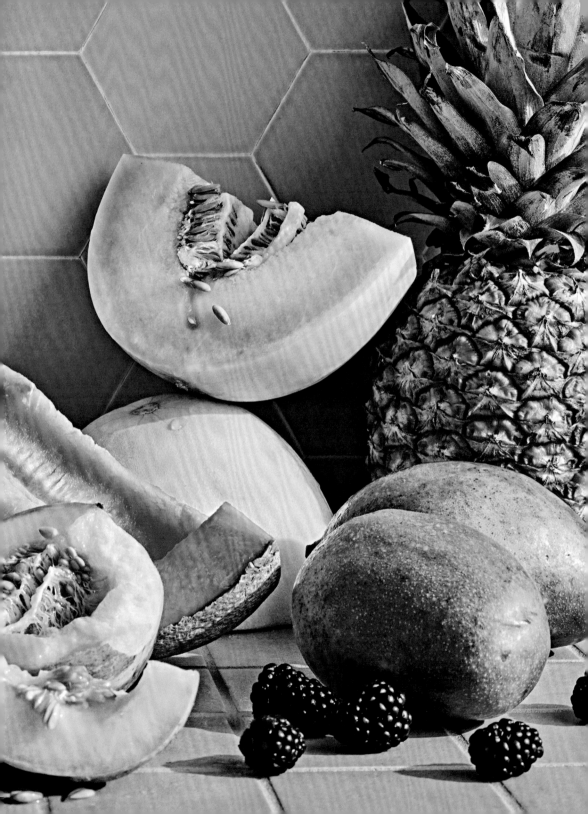

MAUI WAUI MAI TAI

Inspired by the tropical shores of Hawaii (and the iconic Maui Waui strain), this tiki drink brings together all the classic flavors of this beloved cocktail, but with the tasty additions of Cannabis-Infused Grenadine Syrup and orgeat syrup (pronounced "or-ZSA"). Orgeat syrup is an almond syrup with a hint of orange flower water, and it's a must-have ingredient in tiki drinks. To best prepare this drink, you'll want to use crushed ice (see page 21). This cocktail includes two types of rum, and crushed ice provides just the right amount of dilution for the most pleasurable drinking experience.

TARGET DOSE:

2.5 to 3 mg THC | < 1 mg CBD per drink (using Cannabis-Infused Grenadine Syrup, page 56) or your preferred dose (using a commercially made THC/CBD tincture of your choice)

EQUIPMENT:

Shaker tin

Rocks glass

INGREDIENTS:

2¼ ounces (67.5 mL) pineapple juice

1 ounce (30 mL) freshly squeezed orange juice, pulp removed

1 ounce (30 mL) freshly squeezed lime juice

½ ounce (15 mL) white rum

¾ ounce (22 mL) aged rum

½ ounce (15 mL) orgeat syrup

Crushed ice

½ ounce (15 mL) Cannabis-Infused Grenadine Syrup (page 56)

Fresh cannabis leaves, for garnish

Pineapple slice, for garnish

Lime wheel, for garnish

1. Add the pineapple juice, orange juice, lime juice, white rum, aged rum, and orgeat syrup to a cocktail shaker tin. Add ice, top the shaker, and then shake for 10 to 15 seconds or until cold—be careful not to overdilute!

2. Strain into a rocks glass filled with fresh crushed ice, and then top with the Cannabis-Infused Grenadine Syrup. You can leave the grenadine as is or stir to combine.

3. Garnish with fresh cannabis leaves, a pineapple slice, and a lime wheel, and enjoy!

> *Note:* **To make this drink a mocktail, simply skip the rum additions and adjust the juices to your taste preference; then add the rest of the ingredients.**

PASSION FRUIT CAIPIRINHA

The caipirinha is Brazil's national cocktail, made with cachaça, sugar, and fresh lime juice. Cachaça (pronounced kah-SHAH-sah) is a Brazilian spirit made from the sugarcane plant. Unlike rum (another spirit made from sugarcane), cachaça presents fresh and botanical notes, making it a viable spirit to combine with cannabis flavors. This drink tends to be quite high in alcohol, so I recommend micro-dosing the drink with 1 to 2 teaspoons of Cannabis-Infused Sugar. If you're a seasoned cannabis pro and you know your limits when combining alcohol and herbal products, feel free to add more—just as long as the sugar equals 1 tablespoon total. For a boost of flavor, I also love adding just a hint of cold-pressed passion fruit juice, which also enhances the color.

TARGET DOSE:

3 to 4 mg THC | < 1 mg CBD per drink (using Cannabis-Infused Sugar, page 55) or your preferred dose (using a commercially made THC/CBD tincture of your choice)

EQUIPMENT:

Old fashioned glass

Muddler

Bar spoon

INGREDIENTS:

1 small lime, cut into eighths

1 teaspoon Cannabis-Infused Sugar (page 55)

2 teaspoons granulated sugar

¾ ounce (22 mL) passion fruit juice

1¼ ounces (37.5 mL) cachaça

Crushed ice

Lime wheel, for garnish

1. Combine the lime pieces, Cannabis-Infused Sugar, and granulated sugar in the bottom of an old fashioned glass. Begin to muddle until the lime pieces have been thoroughly juiced and combined with the sugar.

2. Add the cachaça and passion fruit juice; gently stir using a bar spoon to slowly dissolve the sugar. You might be stirring for a few minutes, so be prepared!

3. Top the glass with crushed ice, stir again, and then garnish with a lime wheel.

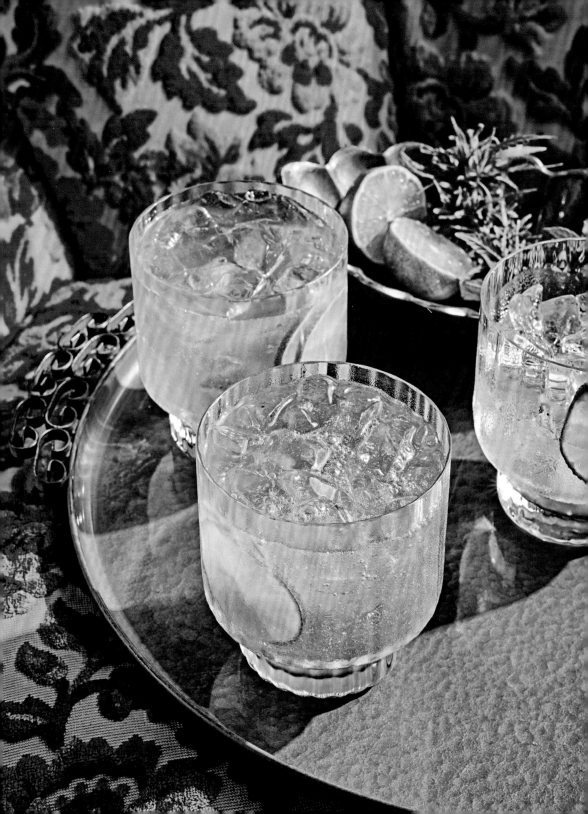

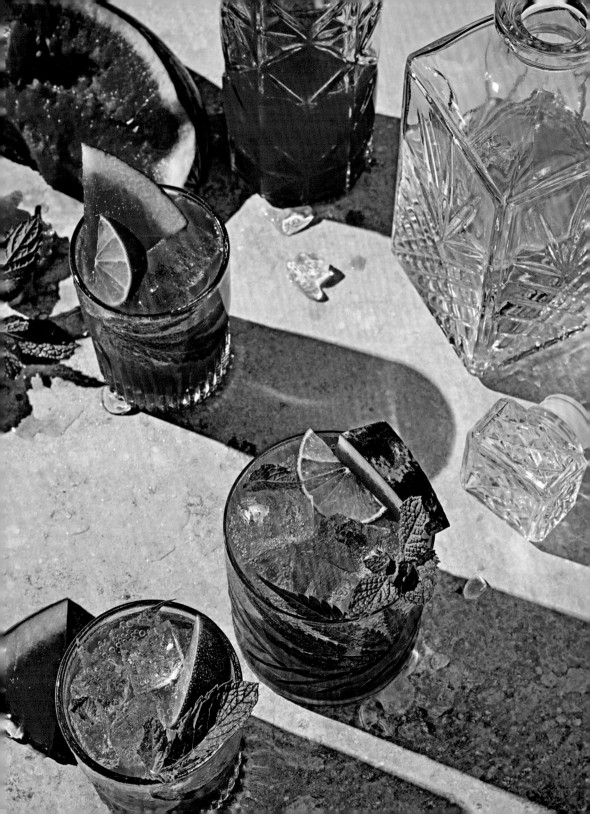

WATERMELON MOJITO

Watermelon is one of the most refreshing treats during the warmer months. Now imagine it in a minty mojito—yes, please! Watermelon juice stays fresh for only a couple days, so be sure to take full advantage of this recipe: Share it with your friends, or enjoy it anytime you're craving something to reinvigorate your taste buds!

TARGET DOSE:

8 mg THC | < 1 mg CBD per drink (using the Cannabis-Infused Simple Syrup, page 49) or your preferred dose (using a commercially made THC/CBD tincture of your choice)

EQUIPMENT:

Blender or food processor

Fine-mesh strainer

16-ounce (480 mL) clean mason jar

Highball glass (or two rocks glasses for a lower dose)

Muddler

Bar spoon

INGREDIENTS:

½ small seedless watermelon (this yields about 1 cup, so save the extra juice for more drinks or make one for a friend!)

1¼ ounces (37.5 mL) freshly squeezed lime juice

5 to 6 fresh mint leaves

½ ounce (15 mL) Cannabis-Infused Simple Syrup (page 49)

1 fresh cannabis leaf

Cracked ice

2½ ounces (75 mL) fresh watermelon juice

1 ounce (30 mL) white rum

Club soda

Slice of watermelon, for garnish

Lime wedge, for garnish

1. Cut the watermelon in half, and add the watermelon flesh to a blender or food processor. Purée for 1 minute or until the watermelon chunks turn into juice.

2. Using a fine-mesh strainer, separate the pulp from the juice over a 16-ounce (480 mL) mason jar (save the extra juice to make more drinks). Discard the pulp, and set the mason jar aside.

3. Add the lime juice to the bottom of a highball glass.

4. Smack the mint leaves in your hand to release the aromas, and then add them to the bottom of the glass.

5. Using a muddler, gently muddle the ingredients to release the mint flavors.

6. Add the Cannabis-Infused Simple Syrup, and then muddle again (be careful not to overmuddle and tear the leaves).

7. Carefully line the top of the inside of the glass with a fresh cannabis leaf, and then fill the glass to the top with cracked ice, being careful not to disturb the wrapped leaf.

8. Add 2½ ounces watermelon juice and the rum, and then top with club soda. Stir to combine, and garnish with a slice of watermelon and a lime wedge.

> *Note:* If you'd like to make this drink a mocktail, skip the rum and simply top the drink with additional club soda until the glass is full. Then continue to follow the directions as noted.

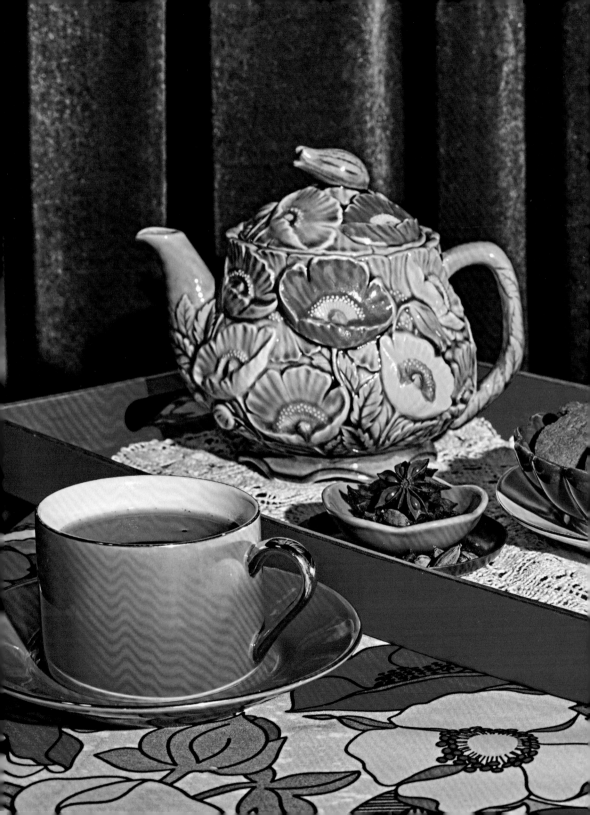

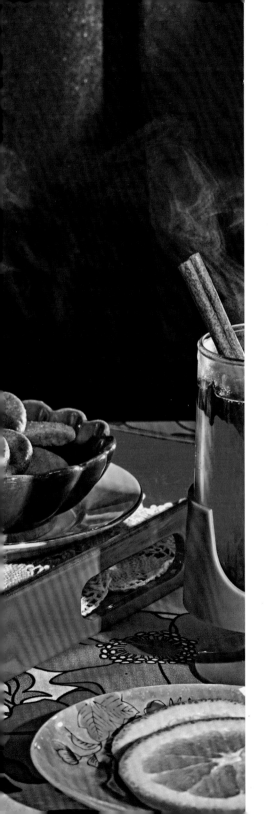

AUTUMN RECIPES

CHAPTER 5

Autumn is one of my favorite seasons because we can highlight so many different spices in food and beverages. Autumn is also when many crops (including cannabis!) are harvested and temperatures begin to cool. It's that special time of year when we can celebrate Mother Nature's bounty and, of course, all things spiced! In this chapter, you learn how to make some of my favorite fall recipes that incorporate classic autumnal ingredients and flavor combinations (think caramel apple, pumpkin spice, and cranberry thyme). Thanksgiving lands in autumn, too, so you'll find some festive recipes to get you in the mood for Turkey Day and beyond. Prepare for a delectable exploration of fall flavors!

HARVEST JUICE

Incorporating some of the best superfoods fall has to offer, this harvest juice provides an abundance of nutrients packed with antioxidants, vitamins, and minerals. Both tart and a little bit sweet, this balanced blend excites the taste buds and will get you in the mood for all things fall! To add a depth of flavor, I recommend infusing this juice with a touch of Cannabis-Infused Maple Syrup; it effortlessly ties together all the ingredients, including the spice notes—plus, it's the perfect enhancement for morning juice!

TARGET DOSE:

4 mg THC | 1.5 mg CBD per drink (using Cannabis-Infused Maple Syrup, page 54) or your preferred dose (using a commercially made THC/CBD tincture of your choice)

EQUIPMENT:

Juicer

Glass of your choice

Bar spoon

INGREDIENTS:

1 chilled Honeycrisp apple, quartered

1 chilled green pear, quartered

⅓ cup fresh whole cranberries

1 chilled lemon, peeled and quartered

2 carrots

One 1-inch piece fresh ginger, peeled and halved (add more if you love fresh ginger notes)

¼ ounce (15 mL) Cannabis-Infused Maple Syrup (page 54)

Pinch of cinnamon

Pinch of nutmeg

1. Feed the apple, pear, cranberries, lemon, carrots, and ginger into a juicer, alternating the ingredients as you continue to juice.

2. Once everything is juiced, pour it into a drinking glass of your choice. Add the Cannabis-Infused Maple Syrup, cinnamon, and nutmeg, and then stir to combine.

3. Enjoy with or without ice—your choice!

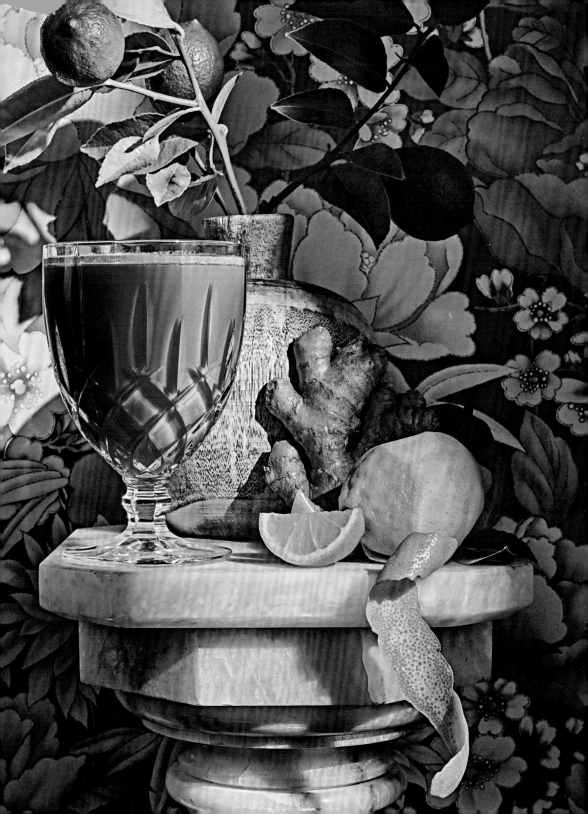

APPLE FRITTER LATTE

Move over, pumpkin spice! This Apple Fritter Latte might become your new fall favorite. Apple butter is easiest to source during fall, but you can still find this ingredient at most grocery stores (or online) other times of the year. It adds both a delightful richness and apple spice notes—yum! To go the extra mile, infuse your milk with the Apple Fritter cannabis strain. It's the perfect pairing!

TARGET DOSE:

5 to 6 mg THC | < 1 mg CBD per drink (using Cannabis-Infused Milk, page 40) or your preferred dose (using a commercially made THC/CBD tincture of your choice)

EQUIPMENT:

Saucepan

Whisk

Milk frother (optional)

Latte cup

Note: **To go the extra mile, create your own caramel sauce (see page 119). If you don't have the supplies to make the Cannabis-Infused Milk, simply skip this ingredient and add your favorite unflavored tincture (at your preferred dose) into the saucepan at step 3, vigorously whisk together the ingredients, and then proceed with the recipe.**

INGREDIENTS:

5 ounces (150 mL) milk of your choice (I prefer 2 percent dairy milk with this recipe)

1 teaspoon apple butter

1½ teaspoons caramel sauce (adjust up or down, depending on your preference—see the accompanying note)

2½ ounces (75 mL) strong brewed coffee

1 ounce (30 mL) spiced apple cider

Pinch of ground cinnamon

Pinch of ground nutmeg

Pinch of ground allspice

½ ounce (15 mL) Cannabis-Infused Milk (page 40)

Whipped cream, for garnish

Caramel sauce, for garnish

1. In a saucepan, combine the milk of your choice with the apple butter and caramel sauce. Begin to warm over medium heat, whisking the apple butter and caramel into the liquid until the caramel fully melts.

2. Add the brewed coffee, apple cider, and spices. Continue to stir until warm (but not boiling).

3. Once heated to your liking, remove from the heat and whisk in the Cannabis-Infused Milk.

4. Blend the ingredients well, creating a slight froth.

5. Pour the Apple Fritter Latte into a latte cup, or use a milk frother to froth the latte even more.

6. If you're a whipped cream lover, feel free to top the latte with a dollop of whipped cream and a drizzle of caramel sauce; then enjoy.

BROWN SUGAR FIG SPRITZ

If you're a fig lover like me, you know that this fruit makes a fantastic pairing with brown sugar, both ideal flavors to highlight during the fall season. Depending on where you live, sourcing fresh figs can be challenging. But during the fall months, they can often be found at your local grocery store. Add a splash of prosecco (or cava), club soda, and a dash of Cannabis-Infused Cardamom Cinnamon Bitters for a delightful autumnal spritz!

TARGET DOSE:

3 to 6 mg THC | < 1 to 1 mg CBD per drink (using Cannabis-Infused Cardamom Cinnamon Bitters, page 44) or your preferred dose (using a commercially made THC/CBD tincture of your choice)

EQUIPMENT:

Medium saucepan

Fine-mesh strainer

Potato masher

Wine glass

Bar spoon

Note: If you'd rather skip the alcohol, substitute with additional club soda. Or, if you prefer a slightly sweeter flavor, substitute with sparkling cider. If using cider, add an additional ¼ to ½ ounce of lemon juice to balance the added sugar.

INGREDIENTS:

2 cups chopped figs, cut into quarters

2 cups water

1⅓ cups (257 g) packed pure cane light brown sugar

1¼ ounces (37.5 mL) brown sugar fig simple syrup

1½ ounces (45 mL) fresh squeezed lemon juice, pulp removed

2 to 3 dashes (or 12 to 24 drops) Cannabis-Infused Cardamom Cinnamon Bitters (page 44)

Cubed ice

3 ounces (90 mL) chilled dry prosecco or cava (see note)

3 ounces (90 mL) club soda (or top with your desired amount)

Fresh figs, for garnish

Sprig of thyme, for garnish

1. In a saucepan, combine the figs and water. Begin to heat until it reaches a slight simmer, then cook for 15 minutes.

2. Once finished, mash the figs using a potato masher, then strain to separate the liquid from the solids. Make sure to double strain if any seeds remain in the liquid, then discard the solids.

3. Add the liquid back into a cleaned saucepan, followed by the brown sugar. Heat the liquid in the saucepan until the brown sugar fully melts into the fig water, creating a syrup. Remove from the heat and let cool; set aside until the next step.

4. In the bottom of a wine glass, combine the brown sugar fig simple syrup, lemon juice, and Cannabis-Infused Bitters. Stir to combine.

5. Add fresh ice cubes, then top with prosecco and club soda. Give the drink a stir using the bar spoon. Garnish with fresh floating figs and a sprig of thyme.

SPICED AUTUMN TEA

With cinnamon, spice, and everything nice, this Spiced Autumn Tea will keep you warm as crisp fall temperatures begin to cool. Celebrating the spiced terpene beta-caryophyllene, which is prevalent in cannabis as well as cinnamon, black pepper, cloves, and many other spices, this tea is packed with antioxidants and soothing properties to comfort the mind, body, and spirit. To infuse this drink, I love adding a splash of Cannabis-Infused Maple Syrup, but feel free to substitute Cannabis-Infused Honey, if it's your preference.

TARGET DOSE:

4 to 8 mg THC | 1 to 3 mg CBD per drink (using Cannabis-Infused Maple Syrup, page 54) or your preferred dose (using a commercially made THC/CBD tincture of your choice)

EQUIPMENT:

Small saucepan

Fine-mesh strainer

Glass mug with handle or mug of your choice

INGREDIENTS:

8 ounces (240 mL) water

1 cinnamon stick

4 whole allspice

1 (1-inch) piece fresh ginger, peeled and chopped into pieces

1 teaspoon orange zest

¼ teaspoon whole black peppercorns

4 whole cloves

5 cracked cardamom pods

1 black tea bag

¼ to ½ ounce (7.5 to 15 mL) Cannabis-Infused Maple Syrup (page 54)—adjust based on your preferred sweetness level

Splash of cream or milk of your choice (optional)

Star anise, for garnish

Cinnamon stick, for garnish

Orange twist, for garnish

1. In a small saucepan, combine the water, cinnamon stick, allspice, ginger, orange zest, peppercorns, cloves, and cardamom pods. Warm over medium heat until the water begins to boil, stirring occasionally. Reduce heat, and simmer for 6 minutes.

2. Remove from heat, and add the black tea bag.

3. Steep the tea for 3 to 4 minutes (or as directed by the tea brand you're using), agitating the tea bag from time to time. Remove and discard the bag.

4. Using a fine-mesh strainer, separate the solids from the liquid over a small mug of your choice; then stir in the Cannabis-Infused Maple Syrup. If you prefer cream or milk with your tea, feel free to add it here.

5. Garnish with a floating star anise, a cinnamon stick, and an orange twist, and serve immediately.

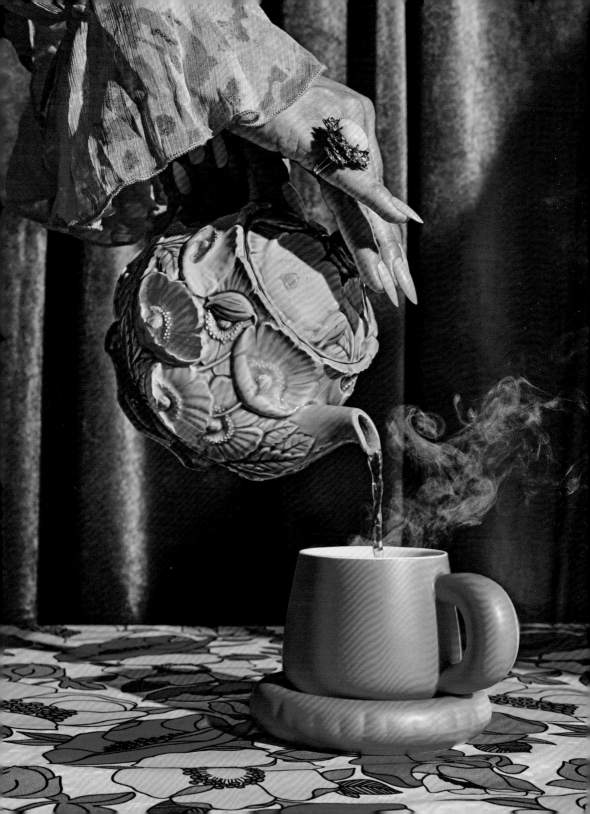

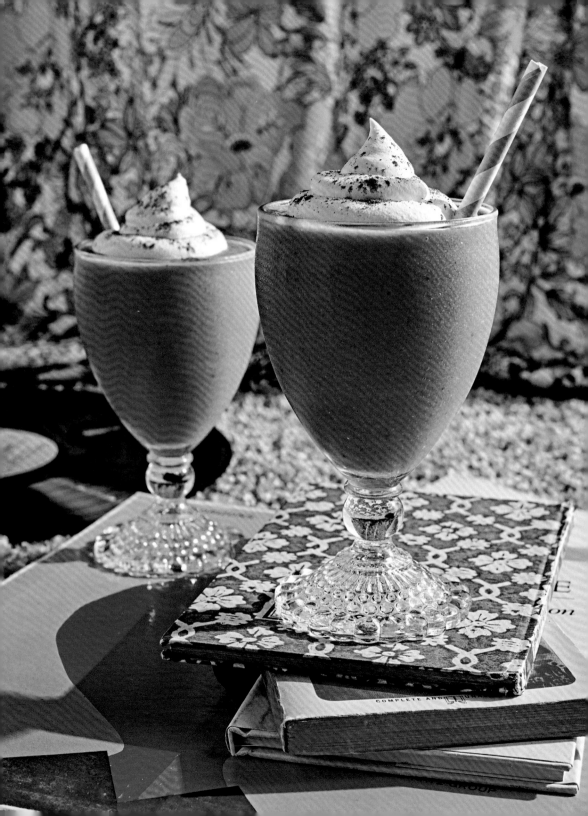

PUMPKIN PIE SHAKE

If you're a fan of pumpkin pie, you're going to love this delicious Pumpkin Pie Shake! Made with pumpkin purée, frozen bananas, the milk of your choice, vanilla protein powder, Cannabis-Infused Honey, and so much more, this scrumptious drink is almost like eating real pumpkin pie—but much healthier. Pumpkin is packed with nutrition, including elevated amounts of beta-carotene, which converts into vitamin A to help strengthen the immune system. It's also rich in vitamins C and E, plus many more nutrients, making it a fall super-food. This recipe is ideal for whenever you have extra pumpkin purée on hand (Thanksgiving time) or whenever you're craving pumpkin pie flavors.

TARGET DOSE:

9 mg THC | 3 mg CBD per drink (using Cannabis-Infused Honey, page 48) or your preferred dose (using a commercially made THC/CBD tincture of your choice—see the accompanying note)

EQUIPMENT:

Blender

Glass of your choice

INGREDIENTS:

⅓ cup chilled pumpkin purée (no flavor additions, just 100 percent pumpkin)

1 cup frozen banana slices

6 ounces (180 mL) milk of your choice (I prefer oat milk with this shake)

1 scoop vanilla protein powder (for creamier flavor)

1 tablespoon vanilla Greek yogurt

¼ teaspoon pumpkin pie spice blend

1 teaspoon Cannabis-Infused Honey (page 48)

1 teaspoon regular honey (or if you want a stronger dose, add 2 teaspoons canna-honey)

Whipped cream, for garnish

Pumpkin pie spice blend, for garnish

1. Add all ingredients to a blender.

2. Blend until smooth and creamy.

3. Serve in a glass of your choice. If you're a whipped cream lover, top with a dollop of whipped cream, followed by a sprinkle of pumpkin pie spice blend.

> *Note:* **If you don't have time to make Cannabis-Infused Honey, you can still incorporate phytocannabinoids into this recipe by adding your favorite unflavored tincture (at your preferred dose) to the blender. Simply blend with the other ingredients, and enjoy. Just be sure to use 2 teaspoons of noninfused honey so the ratios stay the same.**

CRANBERRY THYME MULE

Cranberry and thyme is a festive flavor combination fit for any holiday occasion! This tasty nonalcoholic mule is both refreshing and easy to prepare. To best capture the thyme flavor, I love making a thyme simple syrup, which helps balance the tart cranberry and citrus notes. This recipe is also infused with your Cannabis-Infused Tincture (page 42), blending seamlessly with the other ingredients, including spicy ginger beer. Mix up this drink when you're in the mood for a mule, but with a fall twist!

TARGET DOSE:

4 to 8 mg THC | < 1 to 1 mg CBD per drink (using the Cannabis-Infused Tincture, page 42) or your preferred dose (using a commercially made THC/CBD tincture of your choice)

EQUIPMENT NEEDED:

Saucepan

Airtight container of your choice

16-ounce (480 mL) copper mug

Bar spoon

INGREDIENTS:

1 cup (200 g) granulated sugar

1 cup (240 mL) water

3 to 4 fresh thyme sprigs

3¼ ounces (97.5 mL) unsweetened pure cranberry juice (not from concentrate)

¾ ounce (22 mL) thyme simple syrup (add more if you prefer a sweeter taste)

½ ounce (15 mL) freshly squeezed lime juice

1 to 2 milliliters Cannabis-Infused Tincture (page 42)

Cracked ice

Ginger beer (see "Resources," on page 148, for the brand I use)

Thyme sprig, for garnish

Whole cranberries, for garnish

1. Prepare the thyme simple syrup by adding 1 cup (200 g) granulated sugar and 1 cup (240 mL) water to a small saucepan. Begin to heat over medium heat, constantly stirring until the sugar dissolves into the water. Add the thyme sprigs, and continue to heat for 6 minutes.

2. Remove from heat, cover the saucepan, and steep for 30 minutes to further extract the thyme flavors. Let cool to room temperature, and then transfer into an airtight container.

3. Combine the cranberry juice, thyme simple syrup, lime juice, and Cannabis-Infused Tincture in a copper mug. Stir the ingredients well using a bar spoon.

4. Fill the mug with ice, and top with ginger beer, slowly pouring until the mug is full.

5. Give it a stir, and garnish with a thyme sprig and floating cranberries. For a frosted look, use frozen cranberries for the garnish.

> *Note:* To make this drink a cocktail, simply add your desired amount of vodka to step 1 and follow the directions as noted.

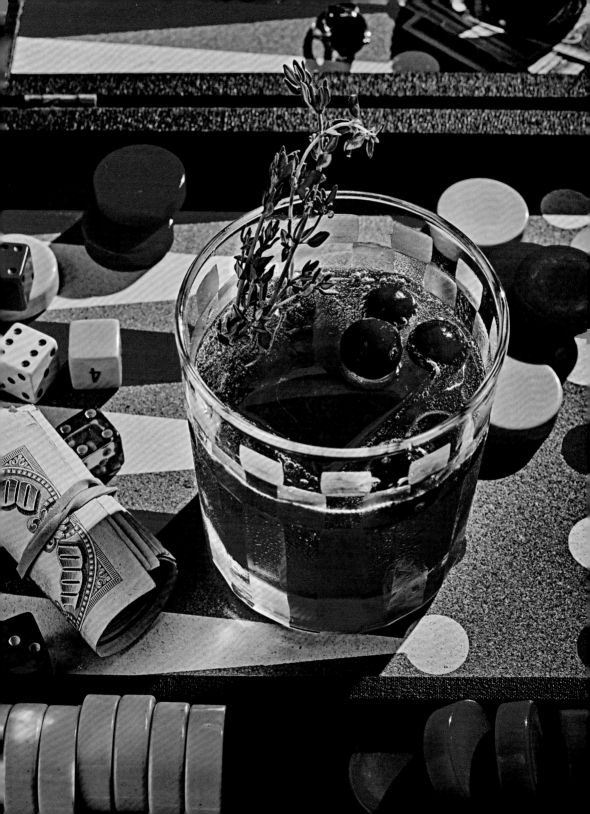

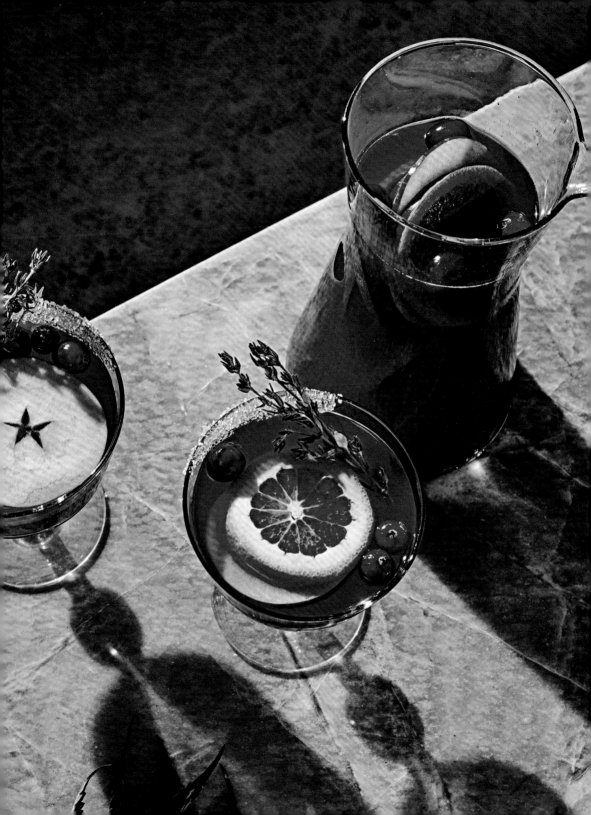

SINSEMILLA SANGRIA

If you're looking to take a break from alcohol, this spirit-free infused sangria is incredibly easy to make and customizable, depending on what autumn fruits you have access to. This recipe serves six people, so I recommend dosing each drink individually using your Cannabis-Infused Tincture (page 42). This strategy allows for a more accurate dose per drink (versus dosing the entire batch at once), to keep everyone happy, healthy, and high!

TARGET DOSE:

4 to 8 mg THC | < 1 to 1 mg CBD per drink (using the Cannabis-Infused Tincture, page 42) or your preferred dose (using a commercially made THC/CBD tincture of your choice)

EQUIPMENT:

Pitcher

Shallow saucer

6 stemless wine glasses

Ladle

Muddler

Bar spoon

INGREDIENTS:

1 orange (cara cara are great for this recipe)

1 small apple

½ cup fresh or frozen whole cranberries

2 cinnamon sticks

1 teaspoon whole allspice

1 teaspoon whole cloves

1 whole nutmeg

32 ounces (4 cups or 1,000 mL) unsweetened pure cranberry juice (not from concentrate)

16 ounces (2 cups or 480 mL) unfiltered apple juice (not from concentrate)

8 ounces (1 cup or 240 mL) orange juice, pulp removed

3 ounces (90 mL) regular maple syrup (add more if you prefer a sweeter taste)

1 to 2 milliliters Cannabis-Infused Tincture per drink (page 42)

Cubed ice (optional)

Thyme sprig, for garnish

Cinnamon stick, for garnish

Cannabis leaves, for garnish (optional)

Orange wedges

1 tablespoon Cannabis-Infused Sugar or granulated sugar—your choice!

1 teaspoon cinnamon

> *Note:* **For this recipe, I prefer to use Honeycrisp apples and Cara Cara red navel oranges because of their unique flavors, but feel free to use your own favorite apple and orange varieties, depending on what's in stock at your local grocery store or farmer's market.**

CONTINUED ON PAGE 118

AUTUMN RECIPES

1. Slice the orange into rounds, leaving the peel on. Core the apple, and slice it into small bite-size pieces. Layer the cranberries and sliced fruit in the bottom of a serving pitcher.

2. Add the cinnamon sticks, allspice, cloves, nutmeg, and juices. Stir to combine. Let the sangria chill in the refrigerator for 4 to 6 hours, stirring occasionally. The longer the sangria rests, the better the flavor will be as the juices and fruits soak in the fall spices.

3. While the sangria is resting, create the cinnamon sugar rim. Combine the Cannabis-Infused Sugar and cinnamon in a shallow saucer. Mix together well using a spoon. If you're serving a group, rim a set of stemless wine glasses with an orange wedge, and then dip the top of each glass into the infused cinnamon sugar blend to create a sugared rim. Set the glasses aside.

4. When you're ready to serve the sangria, use a ladle to scoop out a few pieces of the macerated fruit and spices, and add the fruit to the bottom of each wine glass. To dose this drink as accurately as possible, individually add the Cannabis-Infused Tincture to each glass.

5. Add ice (if using), and then top with the spiced sangria and the remaining macerated fruit.

6. Garnish with a sprig of thyme, a cinnamon stick, and cannabis leaves (optional), and enjoy!

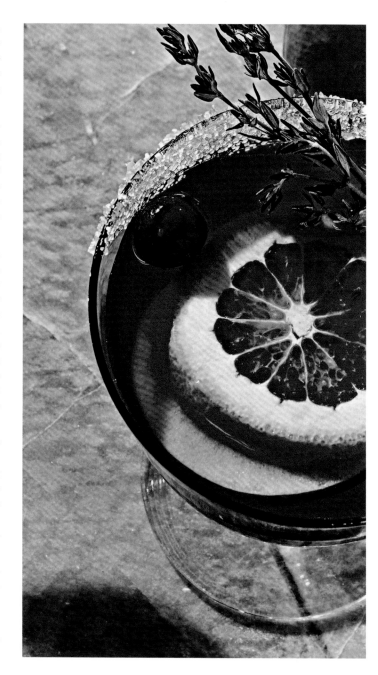

CARAMEL APPLE HOT TODDY

If you haven't made caramel before, don't fret: It's simple to make on the stovetop. Once prepared, you can combine it into several different drinks and desserts (or even eat it with a spoon!), but my preference is to combine it into this seasonal apple-spiced hot toddy. This recipe is so warm and comforting—it's a must-drink on a chilly autumn evening!

TARGET DOSE:

4 mg THC | < 1 mg CBD per drink (using the Cannabis-Infused Tincture, page 42) or your preferred dose

EQUIPMENT:

Small nonstick saucepan

Rubber spatula

Fine-mesh strainer

Warmed mug of your choice

INGREDIENTS:

1 cup (200 g) granulated sugar

2 ounces (60 mL) water (optional, but recommended to reduce risk of burning)

2 tablespoons butter, room temperature

6 ounces (180 mL) heavy cream

¼ teaspoon salt

6 ounces (180 mL) hot water

1¼ ounces (37.5 mL) spiced rum (or whiskey, if you prefer)

2 ounces (60 mL) spiced apple cider

¾ ounce (22 mL) freshly squeezed lemon juice

2 to 3 teaspoons homemade caramel sauce (for a richer caramel flavor, go with 3)

1 milliliter Cannabis-Infused Tincture (page 42)

Apple slice, for garnish

Star anise, for garnish

1. In a small saucepan, heat the granulated sugar and water over medium heat, constantly stirring with a rubber spatula. Continue to stir until the sugar melts and becomes a clear liquid. Turn up the heat, and continue to cook and stir until the caramel turns into a golden-brown syrup. Be careful not to burn it!

2. Add the butter, and stir vigorously into the sugar as it bubbles and melts completely.

3. Turn down the heat, and stir in the heavy cream, continuing to stir. Allow the caramel to bubble and boil for about 45 seconds while vigorously stirring; then reduce the heat again. Stir for 1 more minute until the mixture is smooth.

4. Carefully transfer the caramel to a mason jar or small glass jar to cool. Add the water to a clean saucepan, and begin to heat until the water begins to boil.

5. Remove from the heat. Then stir in the spiced rum, spiced apple cider, lemon juice, caramel sauce, and Cannabis-Infused Tincture. Mix well to combine, and then pour into a warmed mug of your choice.

6. Garnish with an apple slice and a floating star anise.

> *Tip!* When preparing the caramel, you might be tempted to use your Cannabis-Infused Butter (page 39) to create it. This infusion technique can work, but be aware that, when cooking the caramel, temperatures can reach 305° F (151° C) or more, which may burn off phytocannabinoids and terpenes.

POMEGRANATE HIBISCUS SOUR

Both tart and sweet, this mouthwatering pomegranate hibiscus sour is both visually appealing, with its bright red hue, and incredibly flavorsome. For the best flavor, you'll want to source 100 percent pomegranate juice (not from concentrate) and prepare a fresh batch of hibiscus tea, which will be combined into this spirit-free mixed drink. For a pop of flavor, I also love to add Cannabis-Infused Grenadine Syrup (page 56) and a blend of freshly squeezed citrus juices for brightness on the palate. This refreshing fall drink is an excellent nonalcoholic aperitif for entertaining, so be sure to have plenty of sour glasses on hand for serving.

TARGET DOSE:

5 to 6 mg THC | < 1 to 1 mg CBD per drink (using Cannabis-Infused Grenadine Syrup, page 56, and cannabis-infused bitters) or your preferred dose (using a commercially made THC/CBD tincture of your choice)

EQUIPMENT:

Chilled sour glass

Shaker tin

Muddler

Hawthorne strainer

Fine-mesh strainer

INGREDIENTS:

2¼ ounces (67.5 mL) pomegranate juice

1½ ounces (45 mL) hibiscus tea, at room temperature or chilled

¾ ounce (22 mL) freshly squeezed lemon juice

¾ ounce (22 mL) freshly squeezed lime juice

½ ounce (15 mL) Cannabis-Infused Grenadine Syrup (page 56)

Dash of aromatic bitters (see "Resources") or, for an enhancement, 1 dash (6 to 8 drops) cardamom cannabis-infused bitters (page 44)

1 egg white

Dried hibiscus tea leaves, for garnish

Pomegranate seeds, for garnish

1. Chill a sour glass by placing it in the freezer.

2. While the glass is chilling, add the pomegranate juice, hibiscus tea, lemon juice, lime juice, Cannabis-Infused Grenadine Syrup, bitters, and egg white to the bottom of a shaker tin. Cover and dry shake (no ice) for 15 seconds. Add ice, and shake again for 15 seconds or until very cold.

3. Using a Hawthorne strainer, pour over a fine-mesh strainer into the chilled sour glass. Shake the strainer to capture as much froth as possible, filling the glass to the brim.

4. Garnish with floating dried hibiscus leaves and pomegranate seeds.

5. Serve immediately, and enjoy!

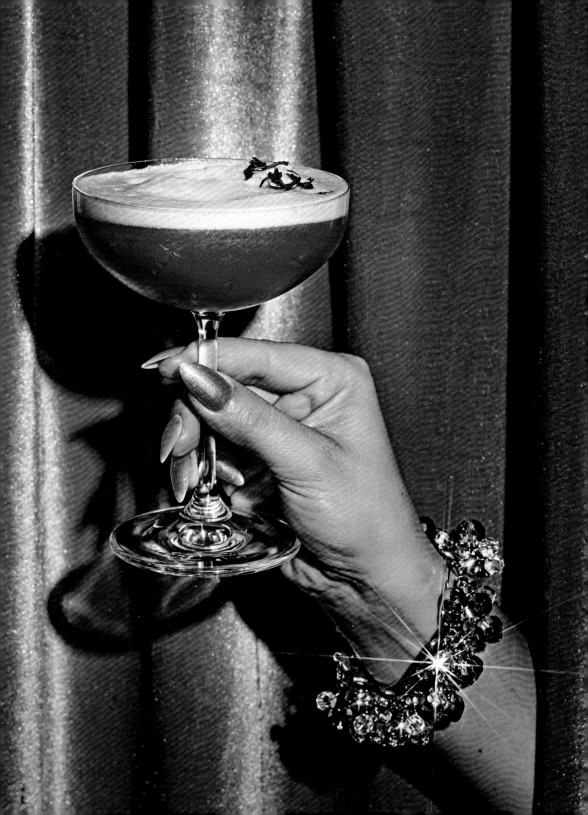

HOT OR COLD SPICED PEAR CIDER

When it comes to fall, apple cider is usually top of mind, but have you ever tasted pear cider? If not, you're in for a treat! This spiced pear cider recipe can be enjoyed either hot or cold, whatever you're in the mood for. It does take some time to prepare (just over 3 hours), but it's absolutely worth making and will fill your house with enchanting spiced smells! Because this recipe yields several servings, make sure to dose each drink individually using Cannabis-Infused Maple Syrup (page 54). It's an instant fall classic!

TARGET DOSE:

4 to 8 mg THC | 1.5 to 3 mg CBD per drink (using Cannabis-Infused Maple Syrup, page 54) or your preferred dose (using a commercially made THC/CBD tincture of your choice)

EQUIPMENT:

Large stock pot

Ladle

Potato masher

Mug

Bar spoon

INGREDIENTS:

8 whole green pears, stemmed, seeded, and quartered

½ whole orange (peel on)

4 cinnamon sticks

6 to 8 whole cracked cardamom pods

1 teaspoon whole allspice

1 teaspoon whole cloves

1 whole nutmeg

½ cup (100 g) packed golden brown sugar

Water

¼ to ½ ounce Cannabis-Infused Maple Syrup per drink (adjust based on your preferred level of sweetness, page 54)

Pear slice, for garnish

Cinnamon stick, for garnish

Star anise, for garnish

1. Add the pears, orange, cinnamon sticks, cardamom pods, allspice, cloves, nutmeg, and golden brown sugar to a large stockpot. Cover with 1 to 2 inches (2.5 to 5 cm) of water, and then bring to a boil. Stir, and then cover the pot. Reduce heat, and simmer for 2 hours.

2. After the 2 hours are up, use a ladle to remove and discard the orange. Carefully mash the pears with a potato masher; then simmer the cider uncovered for another hour.

3. Strain the liquid through a fine-mesh strainer into a clean saucepan or pitcher. Add the Cannabis-Infused Maple Syrup to each mug, and top with the warmed pear cider. Stir to combine; garnish with a pear slice, cinnamon stick, and floating star anise.

> *Note:* This drink can also be enjoyed cold. Simply let the pear cider chill to room temperature, and then combine it with Cannabis-Infused Maple Syrup. Stir to thoroughly combine, pour over ice, and garnish with a pear slice. Enjoy!

MAPLE OLD FASHIONED

For old fashioned fans, this decadent cannabis-infused Maple Syrup Old Fashioned recipe might become a new autumn favorite! Incorporating all the traditional ingredients, but with a twist, this easy-to-make canna-cocktail is a crowd-pleaser and will make you salivate with its rich, opulent flavors. For an enhancement, add a dash of the cardamom cannabis-infused bitters to heighten the flavor, and serve over one large ice cube for the best dilution.

TARGET DOSE:

4 to 7 mg THC | 1.5 to 2 mg CBD per drink (using Cannabis-Infused Maple Syrup, page 54, and the cardamom cannabis-infused bitters, page 44) or your preferred dose (using a commercially made alcohol THC/CBD tincture of your choice)

EQUIPMENT:

Mixing glass

Bar spoon

Old fashioned glass

INGREDIENTS:

2 ounces (60 mL) rye whiskey

¼ ounce (7.5 mL) Cannabis-Infused Maple Syrup (page 54)

2 dashes aromatic bitters (flip to "Resources" for my favorite)—or, for an enhancement, add 1 dash cardamom cannabis-infused bitters (page 44) and 1 dash aromatic bitters

1 large ice cube

Orange twist, for garnish

1. In a mixing glass, combine the rye whiskey, Cannabis-Infused Maple Syrup, and bitters. Stir using a bar spoon, add ice, and then stir again until the liquid is thoroughly chilled.

2. Place one large ice cube into an old fashioned glass. Strain the liquid into the glass.

3. Express the oil of the orange rind over the glass, and then garnish with the orange twist.

> *Note:* This cocktail is high in alcohol, so I recommend sticking to a low dose of THC. If you'd rather skip the alcohol altogether, you can still prepare this recipe using a nonalcoholic bourbon or a cannabis-infused spirit that mimics bourbon notes (just be sure to swap for plain maple syrup).

APPLE CIDER SMASH

When it comes to fall, nothing is more satisfying than apple cider to get you in the cozy autumnal mood. For an adult enhancement, apple cider can be combined with bourbon and cannabis-infused ingredients to create an even better seasonal drink! Meet the Apple Cider Smash. This tasty canna-cocktail is a spin on the classic Whiskey Smash, with a few special ingredients to excite the palate, including spiced apple cider and Cannabis-Infused Simple Syrup. Mix up this easy-to-make recipe the next time you're dreaming about apple cider, but with a twist!

TARGET DOSE:

8 mg THC | < 1 mg CBD per drink (using Cannabis-Infused Simple Syrup, page 49) or your preferred dose (using a commercially made THC/CBD tincture of your choice)

EQUIPMENT:

Saucer

Spoon

Old fashioned glass

Shaker tin

Muddler

Hawthorne strainer

Fine-mesh strainer

INGREDIENTS:

1 teaspoon granulated sugar

¼ teaspoon cinnamon

Lemon wedge

3 lemon wedges

5 to 6 fresh mint leaves

1¾ ounces (52 mL) bourbon

½ ounce (15 mL) Cannabis-Infused Simple Syrup (page 49)

3 ounces (90 mL) spiced apple cider

Crushed ice

Apple slice, for garnish

Mint sprig, for garnish

Cinnamon stick, for garnish

1. Begin by creating the cinnamon sugar rim.

2. Combine the sugar and cinnamon in a shallow saucer. Mix together well using a spoon. Rim a rocks glass with a lemon wedge, and then dip the top of the glass into the cinnamon sugar blend to create a sugared rim. Set aside.

3. Smack the mint leaves to release the aromas, and then add them to the bottom of a shaker tin along with the lemon wedges. Using a muddler, muddle the lemon and mint to best extract the juice and oils from the peel and leaves.

4. Add the bourbon, Cannabis-Infused Simple Syrup, and apple cider to the shaker tin. Add ice, cover the shaker, and then shake until cold.

5. Using a Hawthorne strainer, double-strain the liquid by pouring it through a fine-mesh strainer into the rimmed old fashioned glass, then top with crushed ice. Garnish with an apple slice, a mint sprig, and a cinnamon stick.

> *Note:* **If you'd rather skip the alcohol, you can still prepare this recipe using a nonalcoholic bourbon.**

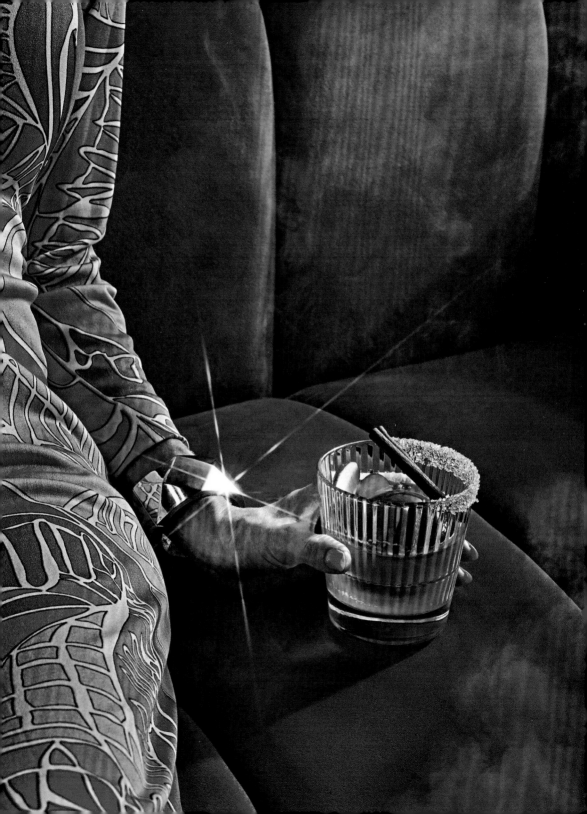

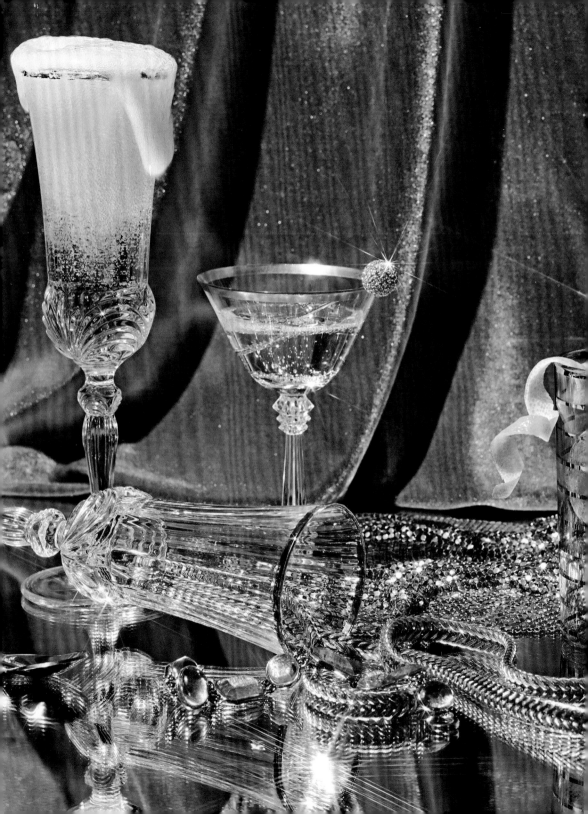

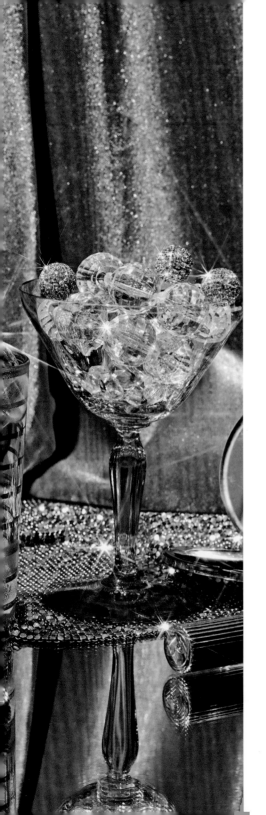

WINTER RECIPES

CHAPTER 6

Winter is the season when we get to celebrate the holidays with family and friends, and warm and cozy drinks are perfect for winter festivities. Sourcing fresh fruits, herbs, and vegetables can get a little tricky during winter, so this chapter focuses on the most bountiful ingredients you can find during the colder months, especially citrus. During the holidays, we can also treat ourselves to some sweeter indulgences, so you'll find a collection of jolly drinks to ring in this joyful time of year!

TANGIE IMMUNITY TONIC

Our bodies need vitamins and nutrients to stay healthy during flu season. Inspired by the iconic Tangie strain (which is one of my personal favorites), this citrusy tonic shot helps boost the immune system with vitamin C and gains anti-inflammatory properties and anti-oxidants from fresh ginger and turmeric. This drink is best enjoyed anytime you're feeling sluggish and need a vigorous boost!

TARGET DOSE:

4 mg THC | < 1 mg CBD per milliliter per drink (using the Cannabis-Infused Tincture, page 42) or your preferred dose (using a commercially made THC/CBD tincture of your choice)

EQUIPMENT:

Juicer

Spoon

Glass of your choice (share or enjoy as an immunity shot)

INGREDIENTS:

1 chilled orange, peeled and quartered (or, if you can find them, substitute with 2 to 3 fresh tangerines)

1 chilled lemon, peeled and quartered

¼ cup chopped fresh turmeric, peeled

⅛ cup chopped fresh ginger, peeled

1 milliliter Cannabis-Infused Tincture, page 42

1 to 1½ teaspoons blue agave syrup (optional, add more if you prefer a sweeter tonic)

Cubed ice (optional)

1. Feed the orange, lemon, ginger, and turmeric into a juicer, alternating the ingredients as you continue to juice.

2. When everything is juiced, stir to combine; then add the Cannabis-Infused Tincture and blue agave syrup (if using). Vigorously stir together, and then pour into a glass of your choice. You can either drink it as is, serve it over ice, or enjoy it as an immunity shot.

3. Serve immediately, and enjoy.

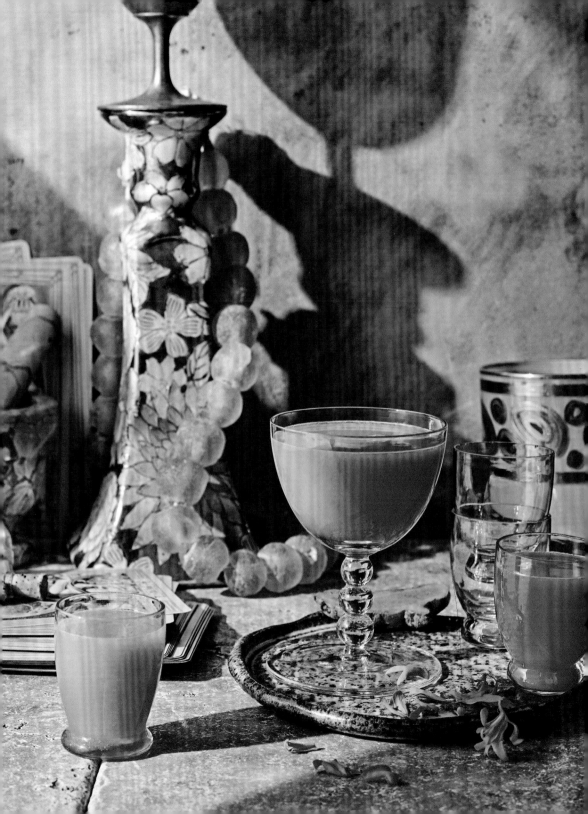

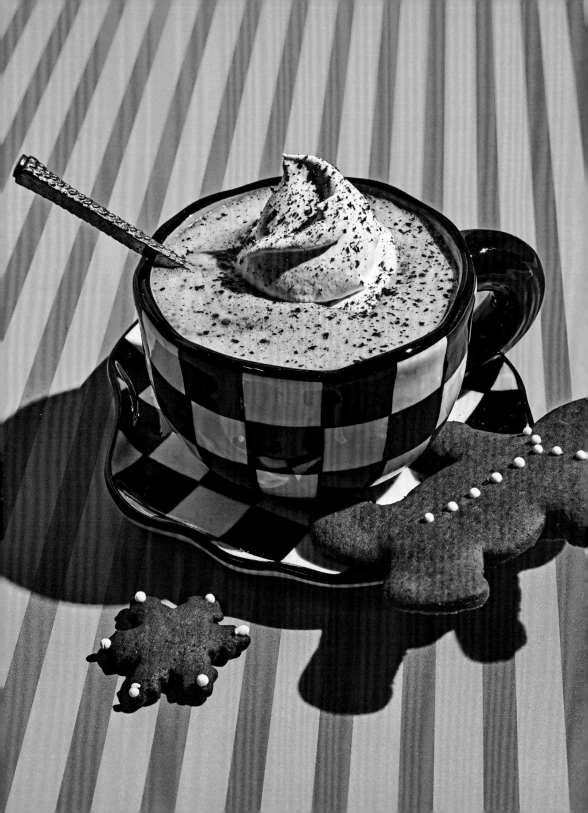

GINGERBREAD LATTE

Sweet as well as spicy, this cozy cannabis-infused Gingerbread Latte is the perfect holi-day drink to enjoy during those chilly winter mornings. Made with the milk of your choice, molasses, ginger, cinnamon, strong coffee (or espresso), and Cannabis-Infused Milk, this decadent latte is the ultimate festive coffee drink you can easily prepare for your family and friends. Add whipped cream and a sprinkle of crushed gingerbread cookies for an extra special treat. You can also dip your gingerbread cookies in the latte!

TARGET DOSE:

5 to 6 mg THC | < 1 mg CBD per drink (using Cannabis-Infused Milk, page 40) or your preferred dose (using a commercially made THC/CBD tincture of your choice—see the accompanying note)

EQUIPMENT:

Small saucepan

Whisk

Milk frother (optional)

Latte cup

INGREDIENTS:

6 ounces (180 mL) milk of your choice (I prefer 2 percent dairy milk with this recipe)

2 teaspoons molasses

¼ teaspoon powdered ginger

¼ teaspoon powdered cinnamon

2 ounces (60 mL) strong brewed coffee or espresso

½ ounce (15 mL) Cannabis-Infused Milk (page 40)

Whipped cream, for garnish

Crushed gingerbread cookies, for garnish

1. In a small saucepan, combine the milk with the molasses, ginger, and cinnamon. Begin to warm over medium heat, whisking until it reaches a low simmer.

2. Reduce heat, add the brewed coffee, and continue to stir.

3. When heated to your liking, remove from heat and whisk in the Cannabis-Infused Milk. Blend the ingredients well, creating a slight froth.

4. Pour the Gingerbread Latte into a latte cup, or use a whisk or milk frother to froth the latte even more.

5. If you're a whipped cream lover, top the latte with a dollop of whipped cream, and then garnish with a sprinkle of crushed gingerbread cookies.

> *Note*: If you don't have the supplies to make the Cannabis-Infused Milk, simply add your favorite unflavored tincture (at your preferred dose) into the saucepan at step 3, whisk the ingredients together, and then proceed with the recipe as noted.

SPICED CANNA-BUTTER TEA

If you've never tasted butter tea before, prepare your taste buds for a delightful journey of creamy goodness! Originating in the Himalayan region, butter tea is typically made with black tea, butter, cream, and sea salt, which creates an almost souplike tea drink. As a spin on this traditional recipe, this spiced canna-butter tea comes together quickly and incorporates chai tea, half-and-half, cardamom, nutmeg, allspice, European butter, and Cannabis-Infused Butter, adding some heightened flavors to satisfy your palate!

TARGET DOSE:

9 mg THC | 1 mg CBD per drink (using Cannabis-Infused Butter, page 39) or your preferred dose (using a commercially made THC/CBD tincture of your choice)

EQUIPMENT:

Small saucepan

Whisk

Mug

INGREDIENTS:

8 ounces (240 mL) water

1 chai tea bag

1 ounce (30 mL) half-and-half

1 teaspoon Cannabis-Infused Butter (page 39)

2½ teaspoons European butter (82 percent milkfat or more)

1 to 2 teaspoons honey

Pinch of sea salt

Pinch of ground cardamom

Pinch of ground nutmeg

Pinch of ground allspice

1. In a small saucepan, begin to heat the water until hot (but not boiling). Remove from heat, add the chai tea bag, cover the pan, and let steep for 4 to 5 minutes, or as directed by the tea brand you're using. Remove and discard the tea bag.

2. Begin to reheat on low. Add the half-and-half, Cannabis-Infused Butter, European butter, honey, sea salt, cardamom, nutmeg, and allspice to the saucepan. Use a whisk to combine well and ensure that the butter is fully melted.

3. Pour the canna-butter tea into the serving mug of your choice, top with a sprinkle of spices, and enjoy!

> *Note:* **This recipe is keto-friendly, supporting a high-fat, low-carb diet!**

WINTER CITRUS SMOOTHIE

Celebrating some of the tastiest citruses the season has to offer, this winter citrus smoothie is just what the doctor ordered! Loaded with vitamin C, flavonoids, and fiber, this power-packed recipe will help boost the immune system while providing antioxidant and anti-inflammatory properties. I especially love blending in freshly squeezed blood orange juice, which adds not only color, but also a hefty amount of anthocyanins, which may help with inflammation. Combined with tangerine juice, pineapple, banana, turmeric, ginger, and Cannabis-Infused Honey, this healthy and filling smoothie is an energizing way to start the day!

TARGET DOSE:

9 mg THC | 3 mg CBD per drink (using Cannabis-Infused Honey, page 48) or your preferred dose (using a commercially made THC/CBD tincture of your choice—see note)

EQUIPMENT:

Blender

Glass of your choice

INGREDIENTS:

4 ounces (120 mL) freshly squeezed blood orange juice

2 ounces (60 mL) freshly squeezed tangerine juice (or orange juice)

1 cup frozen pineapple chunks

1 small frozen banana

¼ teaspoon ground turmeric

¼ teaspoon ground ginger

1 teaspoon Cannabis-Infused Honey (page 48)

1 blood orange slice, for garnish

1. Add all ingredients to a blender.

2. Blend until smooth and creamy.

3. Serve in a glass of your choice, garnished with a blood orange slice.

> *Note:* If you don't have time to make Cannabis-Infused Honey, you can still incorporate phytocannabinoids into this recipe by adding your favorite unflavored tincture (at your preferred dose) to the blender. Simply blend with the other ingredients called for and enjoy. Just be sure to use noninfused honey so the ratios stay the same.

CANNA-CRANBERRY PALOMA

Made with freshly squeezed grapefruit juice, lime juice, cranberry juice, Cannabis-Infused Tincture, agave nectar, tequila, and a splash of club soda, this tasty drink will quickly become a household favorite. Feel free to adjust the blue agave nectar up or down depending on your preference and the sweetness of your grapefruit.

TARGET DOSE:

4 mg THC | < 1 mg CBD per drink (using the Cannabis-Infused Tincture, page 42) or your preferred dose (using a commercially made THC/CBD tincture of your choice)

EQUIPMENT:

Saucer or bowl

Rocks glass

Shaker tin

Hawthorne strainer

Bar spoon

Tip! **To add an extra kick to this recipe, I recommend using Cannabis-Infused Sugar mixed with cinnamon for the rim. Just be sure to let everyone know the rim is infused with THC, to keep the good vibes flowing.**

INGREDIENTS:

1 teaspoon Cannabis-Infused Sugar (page 55)

¼ teaspoon cinnamon

Lime wedge

2½ ounces (75 mL) grapefruit juice (pulp removed)

1 ounce (30 mL) unsweetened pure cranberry juice (not from concentrate)

1 ounce (30 mL) freshly squeezed lime juice

½ ounce (15 mL) blue agave syrup

1 milliliter (or your preferred dose) Cannabis-Infused Tincture (page 42)

1 ounce (30 mL) tequila blanco (optional)

Cubed ice

Splash of Club soda

Grapefruit wedge, for garnish

Frozen whole cranberries, for garnish

Cinnamon stick, for garnish

Rosemary sprig, for garnish

1. Add the Cannabis-Infused Sugar and cinnamon to a shallow saucer or bowl. Rim a portion of the top of the glass with a lime wedge, and then dip the top of the glass into the mixture, creating a partial rim. Set aside.

2. In a shaker tin, add the grapefruit juice, cranberry juice, lime juice, blue agave syrup, Cannabis-Infused Tincture, and tequila. Add ice, and then shake for 15 seconds or until very cold.

3. Carefully strain the liquid into the sugar-rimmed glass filled with fresh ice.

4. Top with a splash of club soda, and gently stir the drink using a bar spoon.

5. Garnish with a grapefruit wedge, floating frozen cranberries, a cinnamon stick, and a rosemary sprig; then enjoy!

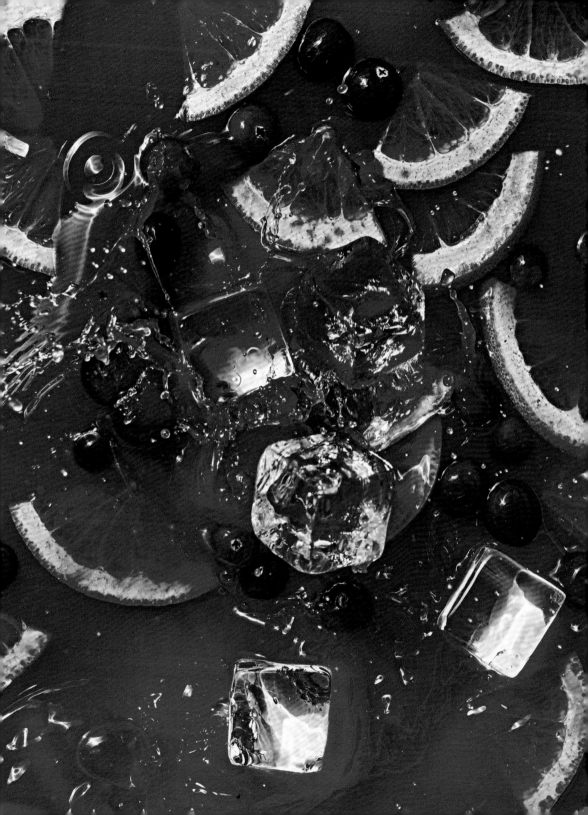

BLOOD ORANGE POMEGRANATE JINGLE GELATIN SHOTS

'Tis the season to celebrate, which means it's the perfect occasion to make some fancy gelatin shots! This time, though, we're infusing them with cannabis. Yippee! This fun recipe is ideal for entertaining and combines the mouthwatering flavors of blood orange, pomegranate, and cherry to honor the festive season. You'll want to have your Cannabis-Infused Tincture on hand to dose each shot individually. Don't forget to garnish with fresh blood orange zest and pomegranate seeds for extra flair.

TARGET DOSE:

4 mg THC | < 1 mg CBD per gelatin shot (using Cannabis-Infused Tincture, page 42) or your preferred dose (using a commercially made THC/CBD tincture of your choice)

EQUIPMENT:

Medium saucepan

Whisk

22 to 24 two-ounce (59.1 mL) shot glasses

Baking tray

Zester

INGREDIENTS:

16 ounces (480 mL) boiling water

8 ounces (240 mL) cold water

2 ounces (60 mL) pomegranate juice

2 ounces (60 mL) freshly squeezed lime juice, pulp removed

2 ounces (60 mL) freshly squeezed blood orange juice, pulp removed (or use cold-pressed juice)

One 6-ounce (170 g) cherry gelatin packet

1 milliliter Cannabis-Infused Tincture per gelatin shot (page 42)

Ginger beer

Blood orange zest, for garnish

Pomegranate seeds, for garnish

1. In a medium saucepan over medium heat, combine the boiling water with the cold water, pomegranate juice, lime juice, and blood orange juice. Stir to combine, and then slowly whisk in the cherry gelatin powder.

2. Continue to stir until the gelatin powder fully dissolves into the liquid.

3. Using 2-ounce shot glasses, add the Cannabis-Infused Tincture to the bottom of each glass. Slowly pour in the gelatin mixture, filling the shots ¾ of the way full (or about 1½ ounces of liquid per shot glass).

4. Top each shot with a splash of ginger beer (about ½ ounce (15 mL), and stir to combine. Place the shot glasses on top of a baking tray, and let chill in the refrigerator overnight or until firm.

5. Once finished, garnish each shot glass with blood orange zest and pomegranate seeds before serving.

CRANBERRY SAGE SPRITZ

This delicious spirit-free mixed drink is a wonderful alternative to alcohol, plus it pairs perfectly with just about everything served during the holidays because it's made with fresh cranberry sauce. Mixed with freshly squeezed lime juice and sparkling club soda, this refreshing bubbly drink will get your palate in the holiday spirit!

TARGET DOSE:

4 to 8 mg THC | < 1 to 1 mg CBD per drink (using the Cannabis-Infused Tincture, page 42) or your preferred dose (using a commercially made THC/CBD tincture of your choice)

EQUIPMENT:

Saucepan

Shaker tin

Hawthorne strainer

Fine-mesh strainer

Rocks glass

Mason jar

INGREDIENTS:

1 cup (240 mL) water

1 cup (200 g) granulated sugar

7 to 8 fresh sage leaves

2 ounces (60 mL) unsweetened pure cranberry juice, not from concentrate (see "Resources," on page 148)

1¼ ounces (37.5 mL) sage simple syrup

1 ounce (30 mL) freshly squeezed lime juice

1 to 2 milliliters (or your preferred dose) Cannabis-Infused Tincture (page 42)

1½ tablespoons cranberry sauce (your favorite recipe, or see the accompanying recipe)

Cubed ice

2 ounces (60 mL) club soda

Fresh whole cranberries, for garnish

Sage leaf, for garnish

1. To make the sage simple syrup, combine the water and sugar in the bottom of a saucepan. Heat on medium-low, stirring continuously until the sugar dissolves completely into the water.

2. Reduce the heat, and add the fresh sage leaves. Simmer for 1 minute; then remove from heat, and allow the leaves to steep for 45 minutes.

3. Remove the leaves, and transfer the sage simple syrup to a mason jar. Store in the refrigerator until thoroughly chilled.

4. When the simple syrup is chilled, add the cranberry juice, sage simple syrup, lime juice, Cannabis-Infused Tincture, and your favorite cranberry sauce to the bottom of a shaker tin. Add ice, cover, and then shake for 15 seconds or until very cold.

CONTINUED ON PAGE 138

5. Using a Hawthorne strainer, pour the liquid through a fine-mesh strainer to double-strain over a rocks glass filled with fresh ice. You want to remove the cranberry seeds and solids; then discard the solids.

6. Top with a splash of club soda, stir the drink using a bar spoon, and garnish with fresh cranberries and a fresh sage leaf.

EQUIPMENT:

Medium saucepan

Rubber spatula

Serving/storage bowl of your choice

INGREDIENTS:

2 ounces (60 mL) orange juice

6 ounces (180 mL) water

⅓ cup (67 g) granulated sugar

10-ounce bag of cranberries

1 strip orange zest

Dash of cinnamon

Dash of nutmeg

Dash of allspice

How to Make Homemade Cranberry Sauce, yield: 6 to 8 servings

During the holiday season, no meal is complete without some delicious homemade cranberry sauce! Whether you eat it as is or combine it into a festive canna-cocktail, here's a quick and easy recipe to try at home.

1. To prepare the cranberry sauce, add the orange juice, water, and sugar to the bottom of a medium saucepan. Begin to heat until the mixture begins to boil and the sugar dissolves.

2. Add the cranberries, orange zest, and a dash of cinnamon, nutmeg, and allspice. Return to a boil, and slowly stir using a rubber spatula. Reduce heat, and cook until most of the cranberries have burst and the liquid reduces (about 10 to 15 minutes, depending on your stovetop).

3. Remove from heat, take out the cinnamon stick, and transfer the sauce to a serving or storage bowl of your choice. Cover and chill until further use.

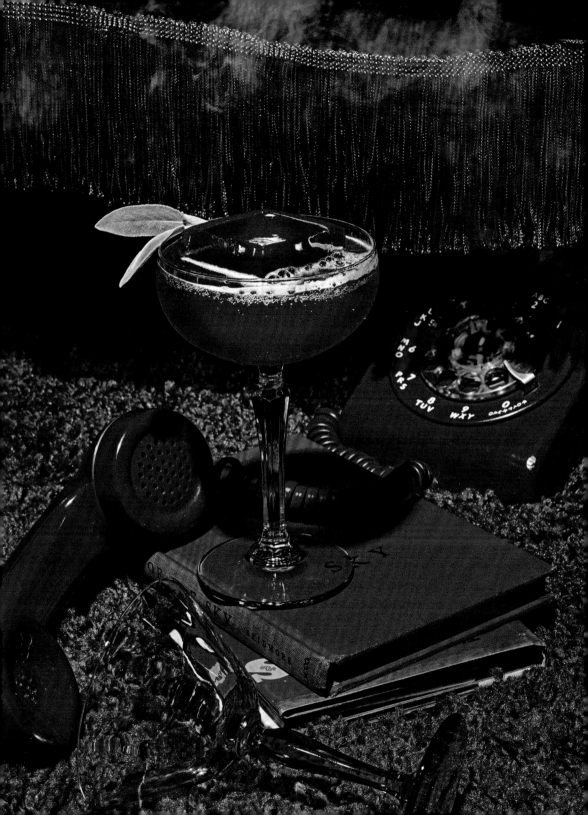

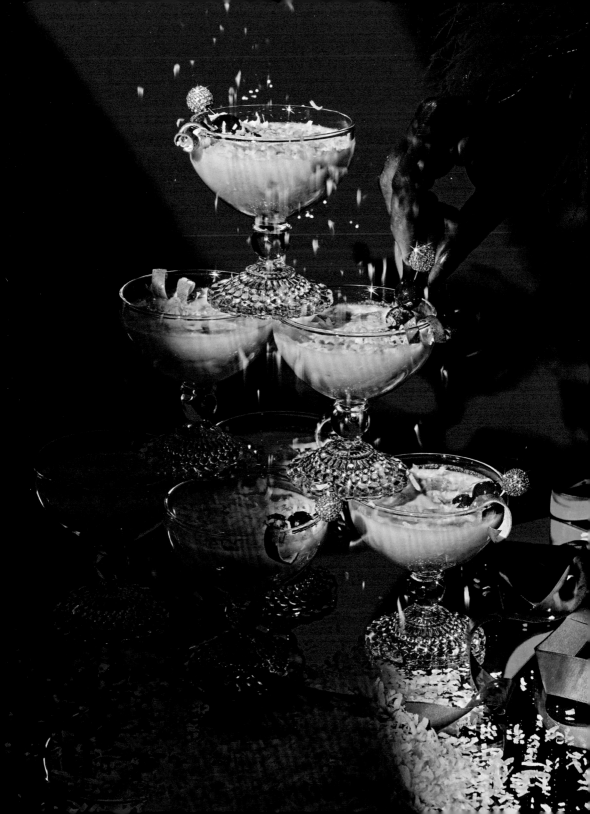

COCONUT CHRISTMAS MARGARITA

Different from your typical Christmas drink, this festive margarita combines coconut milk, cannabis-infused coconut cream, lime juice, reposado tequila, triple sec, and orgeat syrup, delivering an extremely pleasurable drinking experience. The orgeat syrup, an almond syrup with a hint of orange flower water, is the secret ingredient to making this drink extra tasty! I also love using tequila reposado here because it delivers deeper, richer notes than a blanco due to oak aging.

TARGET DOSE:

5 to 6 mg THC | < 1 mg CBD per drink (using Cannabis-Infused Super Creamy Coconut Milk, page 41) or your preferred dose (using a commercially made THC/CBD tincture of your choice)

EQUIPMENT:

Shaker tin

Hawthorne strainer

Rocks glass (or glass of your choice)

Note: **For this recipe, I recommend using a coconut milk that has a more pronounced coconut flavor. If you use a coconut milk that's meant to be refrigerated and won't solidify when chilled, the drink will be smoother and silkier on the palate.**

INGREDIENTS:

3 ounces (90 mL) your favorite coconut milk (see note)

½ ounce (15 mL) Cannabis-Infused Super Creamy Coconut Milk (page 41)

1¾ ounces (52 mL) freshly squeezed lime juice

1¼ ounces (37.5 mL) tequila reposado

¾ ounce (22 mL) triple sec

½ ounce (15 mL) orgeat syrup

Cubed ice

Toasted flaked coconut, for garnish (make sure to use the sweetened kind)

Freshly grated nutmeg, for garnish

Lime twist, for garnish

Whole cranberries, for garnish

Sprig of rosemary (optional), for garnish

1. Combine the coconut milk, Cannabis-Infused Super Creamy Coconut Milk, lime juice, tequila, triple sec, and orgeat syrup in a shaker tin. Add ice, cover, and then shake for 15 seconds or until cold.

2. Using a Hawthorne strainer, strain the liquid into a rimmed rocks glass filled with fresh cubed ice.

3. Garnish with a sprinkle of toasted flaked coconut, freshly grated nutmeg, a lime twist, sprig of rosemary, and floating cranberries.

CANNA-EGGNOG

The holidays wouldn't be the same without some homemade eggnog. But this isn't your average eggnog: It's infused with cannabis—cheers to that! This creamy, rich, and flavorsome drink is perfectly spiced and infused with all the right ingredients. You can also make this recipe with or without alcohol, making it a wonderful addition to any holiday gathering!

TARGET DOSE:

5 to 6 mg THC | < 1 mg CBD per drink (using Cannabis-Infused Milk, page 40) or your preferred dose (using a commercially made THC/CBD tincture of your choice)

EQUIPMENT:

Large mixing bowl

Whisk

Saucepan

Ladle

Fine-mesh strainer

Serving pitcher

Glass of your choice

Bar spoon

INGREDIENTS:

5 large egg yolks

½ cup (100 g) granulated sugar

6 ounces (180 mL) heavy whipping cream

14 ounces (420 mL) milk

½ teaspoon ground nutmeg

¼ teaspoon cinnamon

¼ teaspoon vanilla extract

Dash of salt

½ ounce (15 mL) Cannabis-Infused Milk per drink (page 40)

A splash of your alcohol of choice—brandy, rum, or bourbon (optional)

Freshly grated nutmeg, for garnish

1. In a large mixing bowl, combine the egg yolks and sugar. Whisk together until it becomes creamy, and then set aside.

2. Add the heavy cream, milk, nutmeg, cinnamon, vanilla extract, and dash of salt to a saucepan. Begin to heat as you continue to stir to combine.

3. Bring to a soft simmer (but do not boil!). Once heated, use a ladle to spoon some of the milk mixture into the large mixing bowl containing the eggs and sugar. Continue this process until most of the milk is in the egg bowl; then pour the mixture back into the saucepan.

4. Whisk the eggnog over medium-low heat until it reaches 160°F (71°C); then remove from heat.

5. Pour the eggnog through a fine-mesh strainer into a serving pitcher or container of your choice; then let cool before placing it into the refrigerator to thoroughly chill. At this point, the eggnog will thicken.

6. Once it's chilled, pour the eggnog into the glass of your choice, and add ½ ounce of the Cannabis-Infused Milk. If you'd like to use alcohol, add a splash during this step; then use a bar spoon to stir everything together.

7. Top with freshly grated nutmeg before serving, and enjoy!

Tip! **This recipe yields a thicker-style eggnog. If you prefer a thinner version, add more milk during step 2, and then proceed as noted. You can also add more cannabis-milk during step 6, depending on your dosage preferences.**

Note: **This recipe yields multiple servings, so be sure to dose each drink individually instead of dosing the entire batch at once. This will ensure the most accurate and evenly dosed end results.**

WHITE HOT CHOCOLATE

During winter, there's no better time to indulge your taste buds than with a White Hot Chocolate. This creamy, delicious, and sinfully sweet drink will keep you warm and cozy during this festive time of year. Made with white chocolate and your choice of milk, this drink can easily be infused using a splash of your Cannabis-Infused Milk (page 40). For best results, add a dash of vanilla and a pinch of sea salt to balance the drink's rich flavors. Don't forget to garnish with a dollop of whipped cream and a sprinkle of crushed candy cane!

TARGET DOSE:

5 to 6 mg THC | < 1 mg CBD per drink (using Cannabis-Infused Milk, page 40) or your preferred dose (using a commercially made THC/CBD tincture of your choice)

EQUIPMENT:

Saucepan

Thermometer

Rubber spatula

Whisk

Mug of your choice

INGREDIENTS:

¼ cup white chocolate chips

8 ounces (240 mL) milk of your choice (I prefer 2 percent dairy milk with this recipe)

¼ teaspoon vanilla extract

⅛ teaspoon peppermint extract

Pinch of sea salt

½ ounce (15 mL) Cannabis-Infused Milk (page 40)

Whipped cream, for garnish

Crushed candy cane pieces, for garnish

1. Begin by heating the white chocolate chips in a saucepan. Keep the temperature on low heat, continuously stirring until the chocolate pieces melt completely and no lumps remain.

2. Turn the heat to medium, and slowly whisk in the milk, vanilla extract, peppermint extract, and sea salt. Continue to stir the blend until it reaches 180°F (82°C), or slightly simmering (but do not boil!).

3. Scrape the sides of the saucepan with a rubber spatula, to best combine the melted white chocolate with the liquid ingredients; then use a whisk to blend until it combines. The milk should look smooth and creamy.

4. When blended together well, remove from heat and add the Cannabis-Infused Milk. Whisk to blend; then pour the liquid into a mug of your choice.

5. Garnish with a dollop of whipped cream, and then top with a sprinkle of crushed candy cane pieces. Serve warm, and enjoy.

MULLED CRANBERRY CIDER

Heartwarming and flavorsome, this mulled cranberry cider will keep you warm during the cold winter months. To best prepare this recipe, you'll want to have a slow cooker handy. You'll also need your Cannabis-Infused Maple Syrup to infuse this drink (page 54). If you haven't prepared this infusion yet, you can easily swap for plain maple syrup and your favorite commercially made unflavored tincture and then follow the recipe as noted. This mulled cider is a spirit-free recipe, but feel free to add a splash of brandy or rum if you're feeling a little naughty.

TARGET DOSE:

8 mg THC | 3 mg CBD per drink (using Cannabis-Infused Maple Syrup, page 54) or your preferred dose (using a commercially made THC/CBD tincture of your choice)

EQUIPMENT:

Large saucepan

Ladle

Clear glass coffee mug, or mug of your choice

> *Note:* If this recipe is still too tart for your liking, feel free to add noninfused maple syrup to increase the sweetness without increasing the dosage.

INGREDIENTS:

64 ounces (8 cups or 1,920 mL) unsweetened pure cranberry juice (not from concentrate)

¾ cup (151 g) granulated sugar (you can substitute with brown sugar for a richer flavor)

8 whole cloves

1 whole nutmeg

8 whole allspice

2 star anise

2 cinnamon sticks

½ fresh orange, cut into quarters

½ ounce (15 mL) Cannabis-Infused Maple Syrup per drink (adjust up if you prefer a sweeter flavor and stronger dose)

A splash of your alcohol of your choice—brandy or rum (optional)

Star anise, for garnish

Cinnamon stick, for garnish

Blood orange slices, for garnish

Whole cranberries, for garnish

1. Add the cranberry juice, sugar, cloves, nutmeg, allspice, star anise, cinnamon sticks, and orange pieces into a large saucepan. Cover the saucepan, and then simmer over low heat for 1 hour.

2. When the hour is up, turn off the heat. Ladle the warmed Mulled Cranberry Cider into individual mugs, and then dose each drink using your Cannabis-Infused Maple Syrup. If you'd like to use alcohol, add a splash during this step; then use a bar spoon to stir everything together.

3. Garnish with star anise, a cinnamon stick, blood oranges, and floating cranberries.

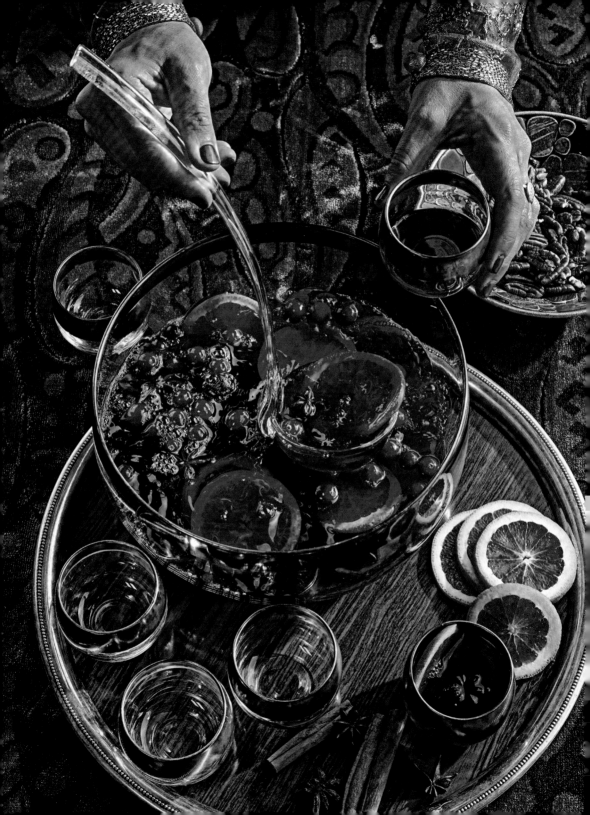

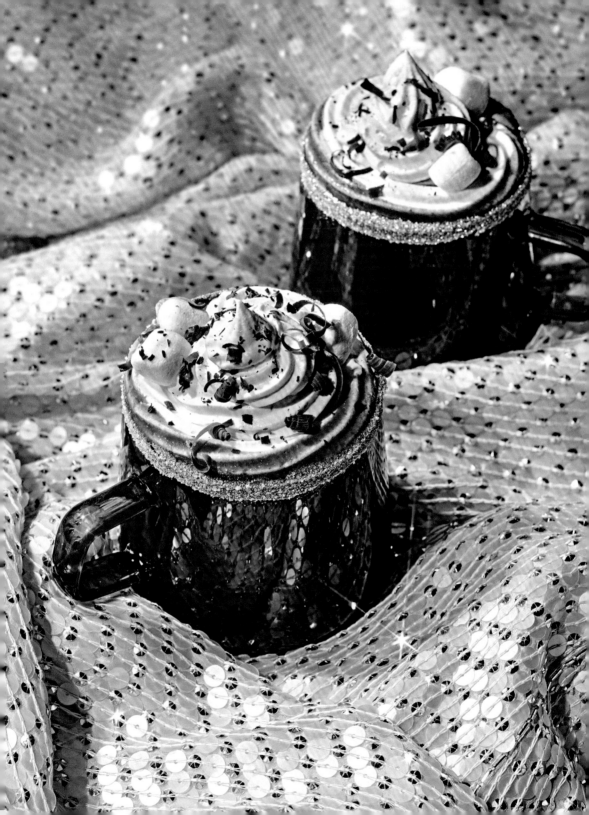

THE STONEY SNOWMAN

Calling all hot chocolate lovers! If you're a fan of the Dirty Snowman cocktail, you're going to love this Stoney Snowman, made with dark chocolate chips, the milk of your choice, Cannabis-Infused Milk, and much more.

TARGET DOSE:

5 to 6 mg THC | < 1 mg CBD per drink (using Cannabis-Infused Milk, page 40) or your preferred dose (using a commercially made THC/CBD tincture of your choice)

EQUIPMENT:

Basting brush

Small saucepan

Measuring cups

Measuring spoons

Rubber spatula

Whisk

Thermometer

Clear glass coffee mug, or mug of your choice

INGREDIENTS:

1 teaspoon chocolate syrup

1 tablespoon white sprinkles

¼ cup dark chocolate chips (I use 72 percent cacao)

8 ounces (240 mL) milk (I prefer 2 percent dairy milk with this recipe, but use what you like)

¼ teaspoon vanilla extract

Pinch of sea salt

½ ounce (15 mL) or your preferred dose Cannabis-Infused Milk (page 40)

¾ ounce (22 mL) Irish cream (optional)

Whipped cream, for garnish

Mini marshmallows, for garnish

Chocolate sprinkles, for garnish

I. Use the tip of a basting brush to paint the chocolate syrup around the top rim of the coffee mug. Roll the top of the mug into the white sprinkles to create a sprinkle rim. Set aside.

2. In a small saucepan, heat the chopped chocolate chips. Keep the temperature on low heat, and continuously stir with a rubber spatula until the chocolate pieces melt completely and no lumps remain.

3. Turn the heat to medium; then slowly whisk in the milk, vanilla extract, and sea salt. Continue to whisk the blend until it reaches 180°F (82°C), or slightly simmering (but do not boil!). Scrape the sides of the saucepan with a rubber spatula, if needed, to capture all the chocolate.

4. When the chocolate has fully melted into the milk and it's mixed well, remove from heat.

5. Add the Cannabis-Infused Milk and Irish cream (if using) to the bottom of the sprinkled mug, and slowly pour the warmed hot chocolate on top.

6. Stir to combine; then garnish with a dollop of whipped cream, mini marshmallows, and a dash of chocolate sprinkles. Serve warm, and enjoy!

> *Note:* If you'd rather skip the alcohol, you can still enjoy the recipe as is! Just follow the directions as noted, and top with a dollop of whipped cream, mini marshmallows, and a dash of chocolate sprinkles.

RESOURCES

Fresh Flower Cuttings
Sonoma Hills Farm

Cannabis Flower
Aloha Humboldt
Moon Made Farms
Alpenglow Farms

Gourmet Pantry Items
Pot d'Huile
Potli
Humboldt Sugar Co.

Ice
Abstract Ice

**Commercially Made
Cannabis Drinks**
Artet Botanical Apéritif
Cann
Ceria Infused Non-
  alcoholic Beer
Herbacée Infused Non-
  alcoholic Wine
Kikoko
Maison Bloom
MXXN Infused Nonalcohlic
  Spirits
Lagunitas HiFi Hops
Wunder

Tinctures
Care By Design
Proof Wellness

**Infusion/Decarboxylation
Devices**
Ardent FX decarboxylation
  & Infusion device
LEVO Infusion device

Infusion Recipes:
Kara Coconut Cream
Peets French Roast Coffee

Beverage Recipes:
*Bitters, Spirits, Liqueurs &
Non-Alcoholic Alternatives
(NA):*
• Amass Riverine (NA)
• Angostura bitters
• Barr Hill Gin (made with
  raw honey)
• Batiste Silver Rum
• Bullet Rye Whiskey
• DHŌS Gin Free (NA)
• Everclear (120 proof)
• Fidencio Mezcal
  Artesanal
• Hendrick's Gin
• La Marca Prosecco Rosé
• Loco Tequila Blanco

• Loft & Bear Artisanal
  Vodka
• JAJA Tequila Reposado
• Modelo Beer
• Seedlip (NA)
• Spiritless Kentucky 74
  (NA)
• Three Sheets Spiced
  Rum

Juices, Club Soda, Other:
• Campbell's Tomato Juice
• Grandma's Jam House
  Strawberry Rhubarb Jam
• Harmless Harvest
  Coconut Water
• Liber & Co. Almond
  Orgeat Syrup
• Open Nature Cranberry
  Juice (Not from
  Concentrate)
• Open Nature Tart
  Cherry Juice (Not from
  Concentrate)
• Q Club Soda
• Q Ginger Beer
• Twinings Green Tea
• Twisted Alchemy Cold
  Pressed Juices (Passion
  Fruit, Blood Orange,
  Pineapple)

WORKS CITED

Aldin, Ben. "What Is Terpinolene and What Does This Cannabis Terpene Do?" Leafly. September 2018.

Bennett, P. "What Is Ocimene and What Does This Cannabis Terpene Do?" Leafly. December 2018.

Bobrow, Warren. *Cannabis Cocktails, Mocktails & Tonics*. Beverly, MA: Quarto Publishing Group USA Inc, 2016.

Booth, J. K., et al. "Terpene Synthases from Cannabis sativa." PLOS One. March 2017.

Chun, H., Evans, J. *High Times: Let's Get Baked! The Official Cannabis Cookbook*. Insight Editions, 2023.

Editors of The Hour. "Ice Matters: 5 Tips for Making Great Cocktails!." The Hour. June 2013.

Evans, J. *Cannabis Drinks: Secrets to Crafting CBD and THC Beverages at Home*. Fair Winds Press of Quarto Publishing Group, 2021.

Evans, J. *The Ultimate Guide to CBD: Explore the World of Cannabidiol*. Fair Winds Pres of Quarto Publishing Group, 2020.

Goldleaf Ltd. *The Cooking Journal: A Cannabis Culinary Companion*. Fairfield, OH: Goldleaf Ltd., 2018.

Korkidis, John. "Fat-Washed Cannabis-Infused Alcohol." Chron Vivant. December 29, 2017.

June-Wells, Mark, Ph.D. "Your Guide to Ethanol Extraction." Cannabis Business Times. 169 July 11, 2018.

Lee, Martin A. "Cannabis Dosing 101." Project CBD. May 2018.

Lee, Martin A. "Terpenes and the 'Entourage Effect'" Project CBD.

Magner, E. "What Really Happens When You Mix CBD and Alcohol." Well+Good. September 28, 2019.

McDonough, E. "Top Tips for Using Hash as a Culinary Ingredient." Leafly. September 2018.

Mudge E. M., et al. "The Terroir of Cannabis: Terpene Metabolomics as a Tool to Understand Cannabis sativa Selections." Planta Medica. July 2019.

ACKNOWLEDGMENTS

I'd like to thank my publisher, Insight Editions, and High Times, for the exciting opportunity to write another book focused on my favorite category, cannabis drinks! This was such a fun (and flavorful) project to work on. Cheers to this fantastic collection of seasonal beverages!

I'd also like to thank my wonderful editor, Sammy Holland, and editorial assistants, Emma Merwin and Sami Alvarado. I couldn't have done this without you! Thank you for supporting my vision.

A heartfelt thank you to my dear friend and mentor, Warren Bobrow, for the continued support and encouragement in this category. Warren, thank you so much for everything and for contributing the foreword to this book.

A special thank you to our amazing photographer and creative genius, Eva Kolenko, and Our House Studio. This was such a groovy and colorful book to bring to life! A big shout out and thank you to Eva, our food stylist, Natalie Drobny, prop stylist and photography assistant, Genesis Vallejo, vintage prop stylist, Kaeja Korty, and onsite food assistants, Paige Arnett and Huxley McCorkle. What a fantastic team and unforgettable photoshoot!

A special thank you to my fabulous friend, Monica Lo, for the headshot, and to Sonoma Hills Farm for the fresh cannabis leaves!

Thank you to my husband, Stratos, for being the best taste tester (I love you!), and thank you to our friend, Donald, for the tasting notes. A special thank you to my family and extended families, The Evanses, The Barbers, The Christianakises, and The vom Dorps, for supporting my work in the cannabis space.

So much gratitude to all of the cannabis trailblazers, activists, and pioneers who have paved the way, and a heartfelt thank you to my wonderful fans and readers who've supported my work from the very beginning. Much love to all. Cheers!

ABOUT THE AUTHOR

Jamie Evans is the founder of The Herb Somm, a culinary-meets-cannabis blog and lifestyle brand that's focused on the gourmet side of the cannabis industry. She's a 4 x author, entrepreneur, and writer specializing in cannabis, beverages, food, wine, and the canna-culinary world.

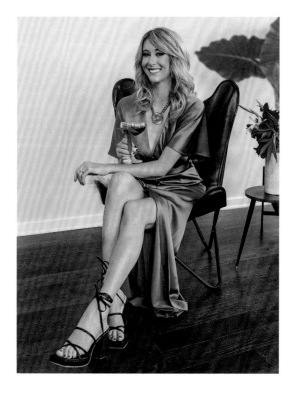

As a well-known cannabis and wine personality, Jamie is best known for her literary work and signature wine and weed experiences. She's contributed to *POPSUGAR*, *Wine Enthusiast Magazine*, *High Times Magazine*, *MARY Magazine*, and *The Clever Root* magazine, specializing in lifestyle features for the modern consumer. In addition, she's the co-editor of GoldLeaf's acclaimed cannabis *Cooking Journal* and author of the published books *The Ultimate Guide to CBD: Explore the World of Cannabidiol* (Fair Winds Press, 2020), *Cannabis Drinks: Secrets to Crafting CBD & THC Beverages at Home* (Fair Winds Press, 2021), and *High Times: Let's Get Baked! The Official Cannabis Cookbook* (Insight Editions, 2023).

As an industry leader, Jamie was named one of *Wine Enthusiast Magazine's* Top 40 Under 40 Tastemakers in 2018 and as a 2018 Innovator by SevenFifty Daily. She was also recognized as one of Green Market Report's "Most Important Women in Weed" in 2020 and named one of Marijuana Venture's Top 40 Under 40 leaders in 2023.

Alongside her work in the cannabis space, Jamie is a Certified Sommelier with over a decade of wine industry experience. She's been featured in dozens of different articles and TV segments, including *Food & Wine*, *Wall Street Journal*, *Entrepreneur*, *Forbes*, *Financial Times*, *Wine Enthusiast*, *Robb Report*, *San Francisco Chronicle*, *Los Angeles Times*, *ABC*, and *High Times*, among many others. Follow Jamie's canna-culinary adventures on Instagram @theherbsomm.

INSIGHT
EDITIONS

PO Box 3088
San Rafael, CA 94912
www.insighteditions.com

Find us on Facebook: www.facebook.com/InsightEditions
Follow us on Instagram: @insighteditions

ISBN: 979-8-88663-379-5

Publisher: Raoul Goff
VP, Co-Publisher: Vanessa Lopez
VP, Creative: Chrissy Kwasnik
VP, Manufacturing: Alix Nicholaeff
VP, Group Managing Editor: Vicki Jaeger
Publishing Director: Jamie Thompson
Designer: Lola Villanueva
Senior Editor: Samantha Holland
Editorial Assistants: Emma Merwin and Sami Alvarado
Managing Editor: Maria Spano
Production Associate: Deena Hashem
Senior Production Manager, Subsidiary Rights: Lina s Palma-Temena

Author Headshot Photographer: Monica Lo

Photographer, Prop Stylist, and Photography Art Direction: Eva Kolenko
Prop Stylist and Photography Assistant: Genesis Vallejo
Food Stylist: Natalie Drobny
Junior Food Assistants and Drink Stylist Assistants: Paige Arnett and Huxley McCorkle
Prop Stylist: Kaeja Korty

Drink Recipes © 2024 Jamie Evans
Terpene Chart © 2024 Jamie Evans

Thank you to Abstract Ice for the ice throughout the book; © 2024 Abstract Ice
Thank you to Sonoma Hills Farm for the cannabis leaves and cuttings used throughout the book; © 2024 Sonoma Hills Farm

ROOTS of PEACE   REPLANTED PAPER

Insight Editions, in association with Roots of Peace, will plant two trees for each tree used in the manufacturing of this book. Roots of Peace is an internationally renowned humanitarian organization dedicated to eradicating land mines worldwide and converting war-torn lands into productive farms and wildlife habitats. Roots of Peace will plant two million fruit and nut trees in Afghanistan and provide farmers there with the skills and support necessary for sustainable land use.

Manufactured in China by Insight Editions

10 9 8 7 6 5 4 3 2 1

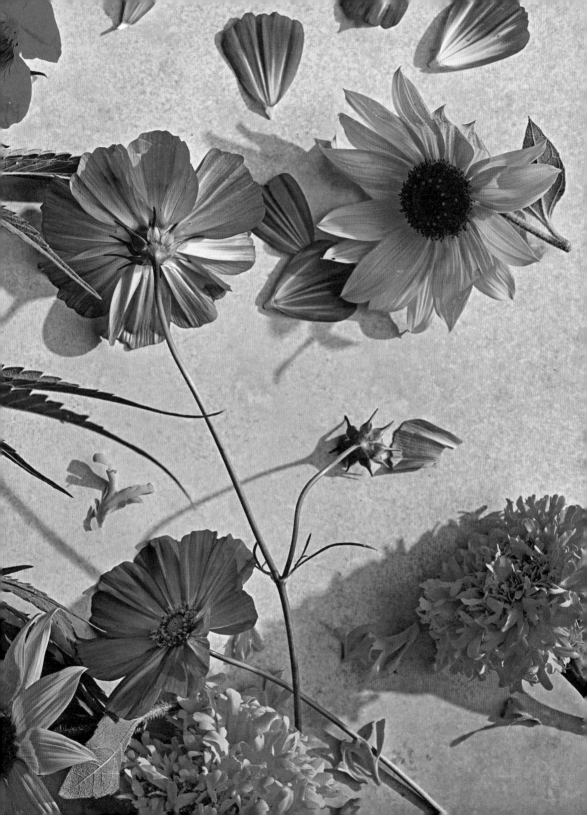

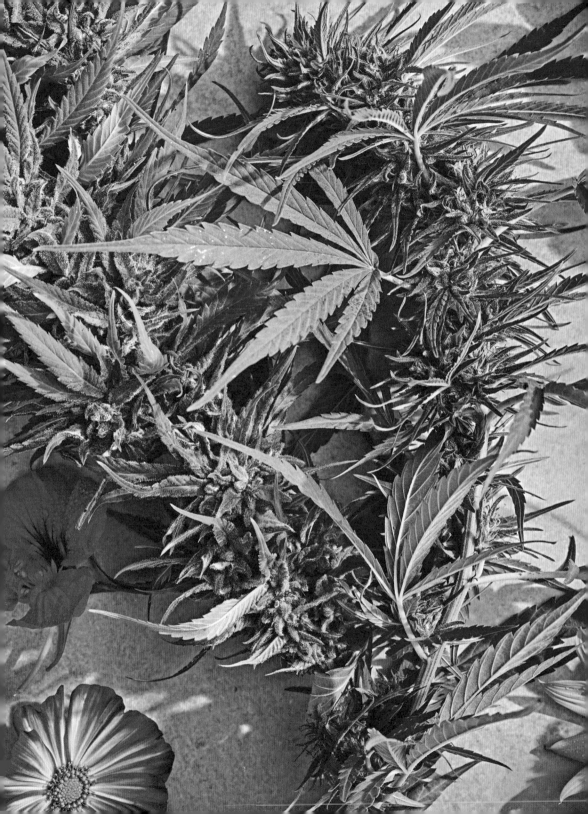